THE

Quit Smoking

COLOURING BOOK

LOST THE PLOT

A Lost the Plot Book, First published in 2017 by Pantera Press Pty Limited www.PanteraPress.com

Please send all permission queries to:
Pantera Press, P.O. Box 1989 Neutral Bay, NSW 2089 Australia or info@PanteraPress.com

A Cataloguing-in-Publication entry for this book is available from the National Library of Australia.

ISBN 978-1-921997-97-6 (Paperback)
Cover and Internal Design: Aga Makowiecka
Illustrations: Yjulia Gramotneva

THE
Quit Smoking
COLOURING BOOK

LOST
THE
PLOT

Cigarettes are killers
that travel in packs

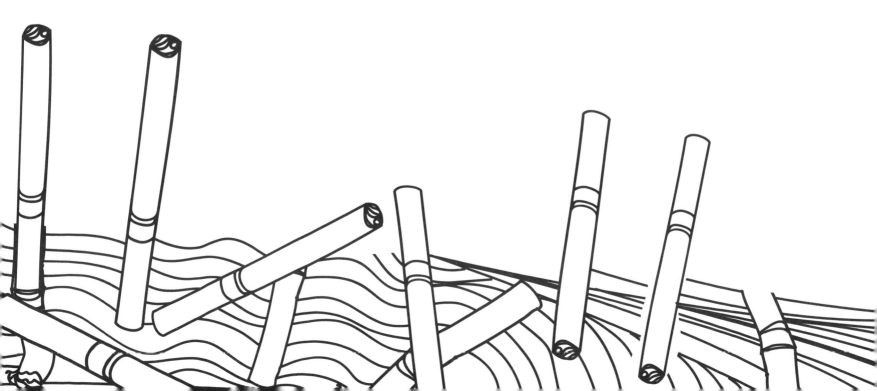

Time

It's estimated that it takes six minutes to smoke a cigarette - it surely doesn't the way you suck 'em down, you animal, but if we count all the time you spend coughing and crying it probably evens out.

At a pack a day, that's two hours every day you spend smoking and doing fuck all else.

Sure, if you've got the world's busiest social life you can justify it saying that you've spent that time spitting some bull with your buddies - but let's face it, all your friends have quit smoking and not as many people are willing to stand around with you doing nothing as they used to.

We both know you smoke more than one pack a day - at two packs a day you waste 7200 hours in 5 years. You could be 72% of the way there to mastering the concert piano, but all you can do is stand out in the cold complaining bitterly. And that's not to mention the 40 years you might save!

Think about all the wonderful stuff you don't have time for that you always want to do, like pursuing your real passion instead of your stupid dead end boring job.

Drop the darts and get on with it.

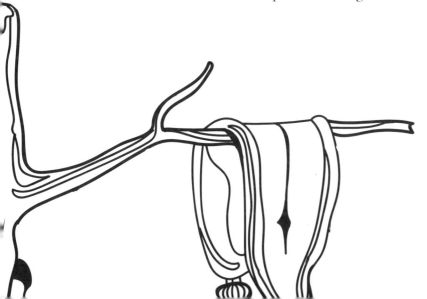

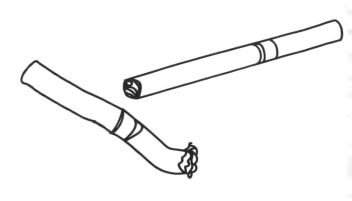

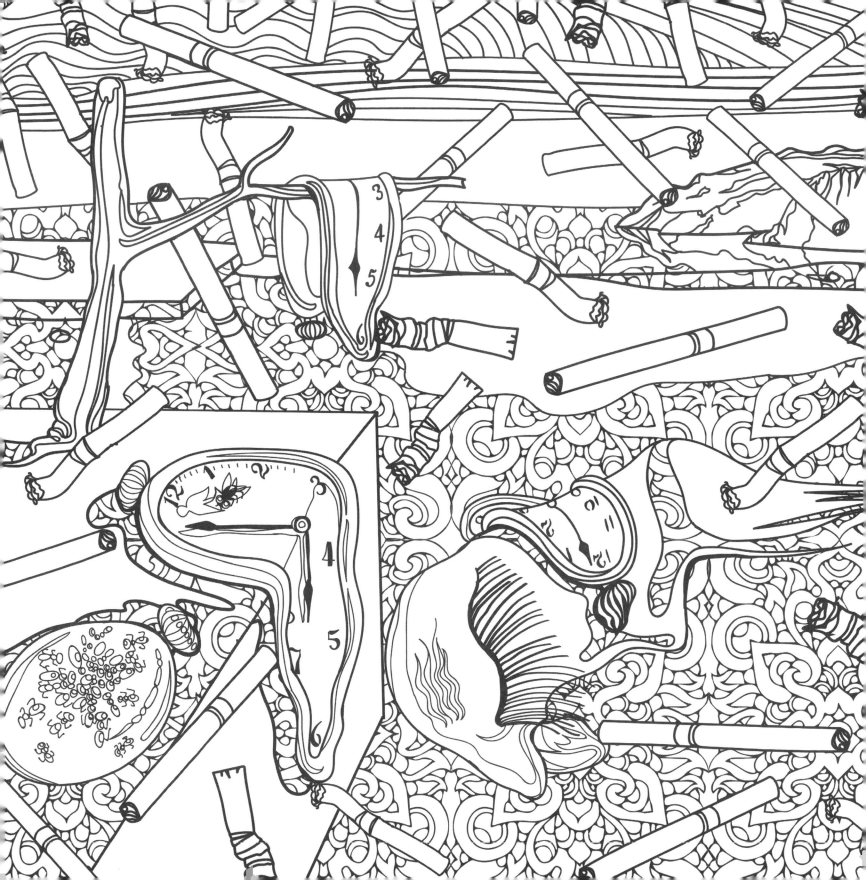

Smoking and homework

Nicotine is a mind-altering chemical and can have beneficial effects - it can calm you down when you're stressed and it can keep you alert when you're tired. This really makes smoking the ideal drug for getting work done when you're on a deadline. Got to pull an all-nighter? Pull out the ciggies and get down to it!

The thing is, maybe you wouldn't be so goddamn tired all the time if your arteries weren't clogged, and your lungs hadn't been destroyed and maybe you wouldn't be so goddamn stressed if you just knew how to breathe!

Just like the car, this is another filthy habit it's time to drop - and think of your poor laptop!

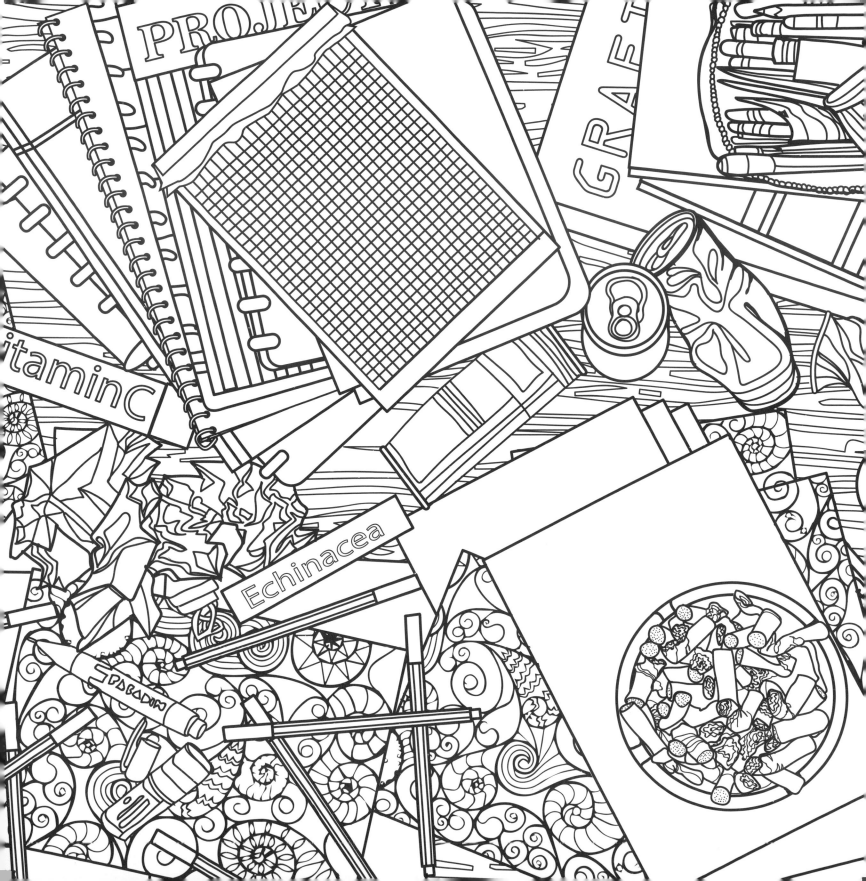

Drinking and smoking

You might argue that there is nothing in your life that comes close to the ecstasy of drinking and smoking - this is probably because you're a fat, smelly loser, but that's beside the point.

What you really need to know is what happens after your evening of debauchery is finished and you wake up with that splitting headache and a mouth that feels like a trash can filled with feral animals that have been lit on fire and dumped by that twisted sicko that lives down the road.

Here is an interesting fact: if you don't have a single cigarette during a night on the town, your hangover will be dramatically improved - you won't even know you've had one.

Those days of lying on the floor, crying watching reruns of shows you don't like and screaming and whining at your friends and family can be over!

And remember this, those non-smokers that complain about how hungover they are - they don't have a goddamn clue.

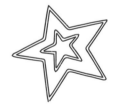

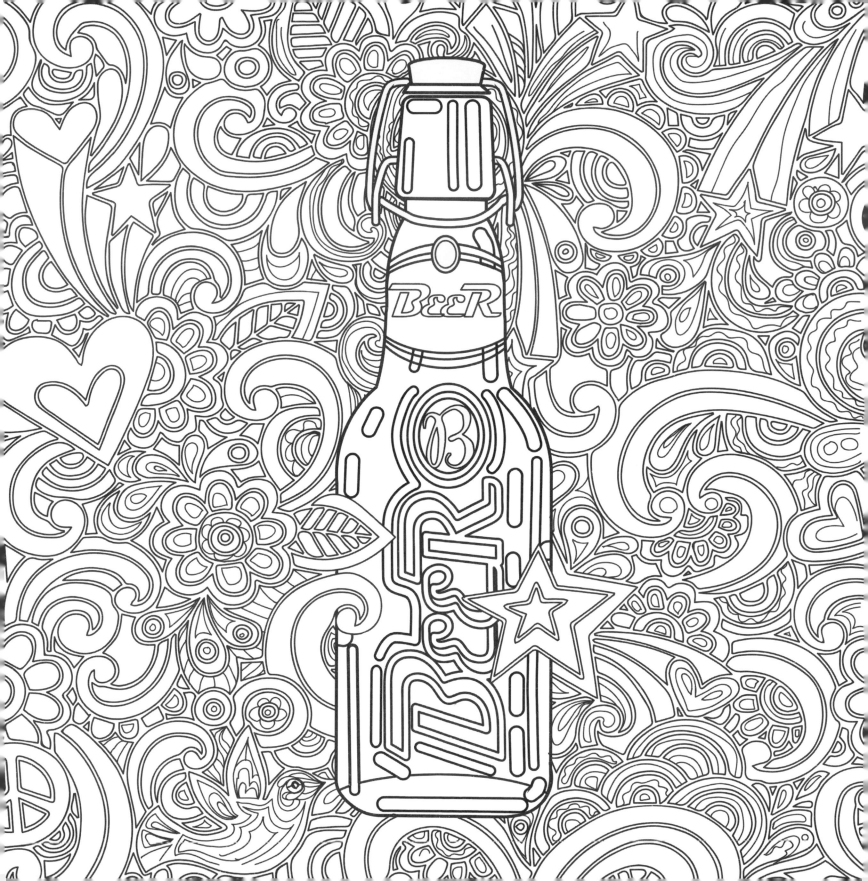

Kickin' back smokin' on the job

Hey, no complaints here - sometimes when work gets to be a bit much you've just gotta kick back.

You still smell absolutely awful, though.

Oxygen has the same calming affect.

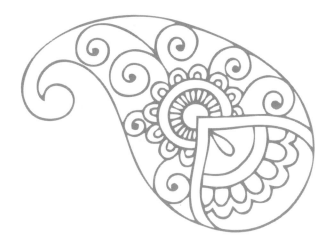

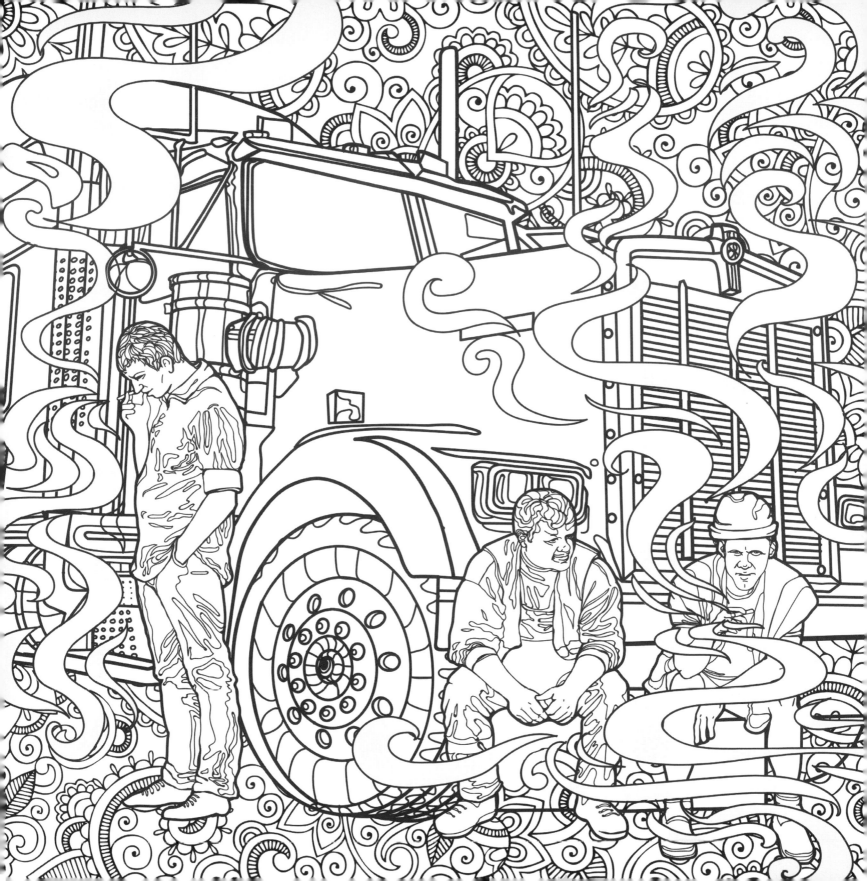

Look at these beautiful bastards

Look again, and then take a real long hard look at yourself.

Your skin doesn't look like that.

You don't feel happy like they do.

No one that looks like them has ever even spoken to you.

You know for sure they don't smoke.

They'll spend the night together wining, dining and having fun and in the morning wake up like it's an absolute breeze and do it all again.

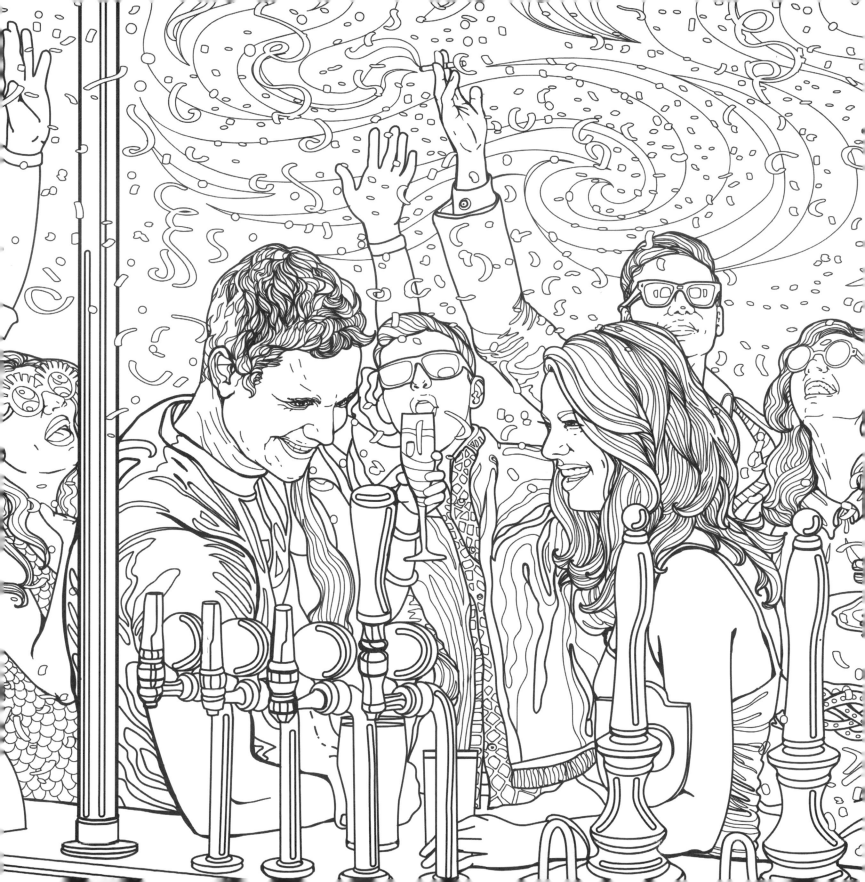

But what about all the beauty I'll miss out on?

It is a myth that you can only go with a friend or two to a beautiful view if you're *all* going to have a cigarette.

You may be worried that by giving up smoking, you'll be giving this up - one of the real treats in your life. But rest assured, you can still totally do this!

And you know what else? At a big group dinner when it's all feeling a bit much and you want to go outside - you can go outside and go grab a breath of delicious fresh air. No one will think differently of you!

The things you think you love about cigarettes aren't about cigarettes at all - you just smoke all the damn time.

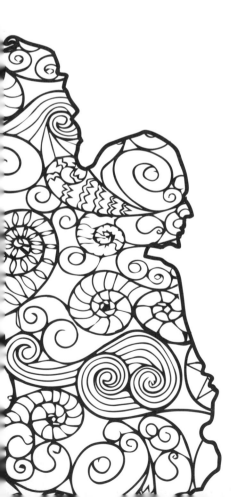

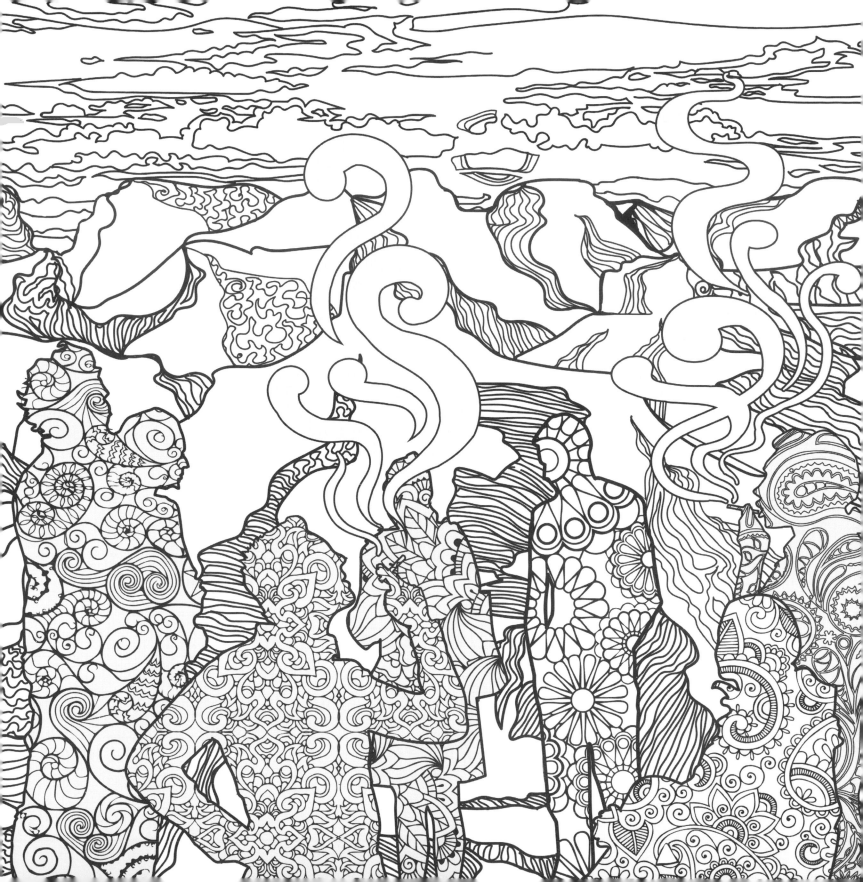

Look at these dogs ha ha ha

They are all smoking and playing poker.
How hilarious.

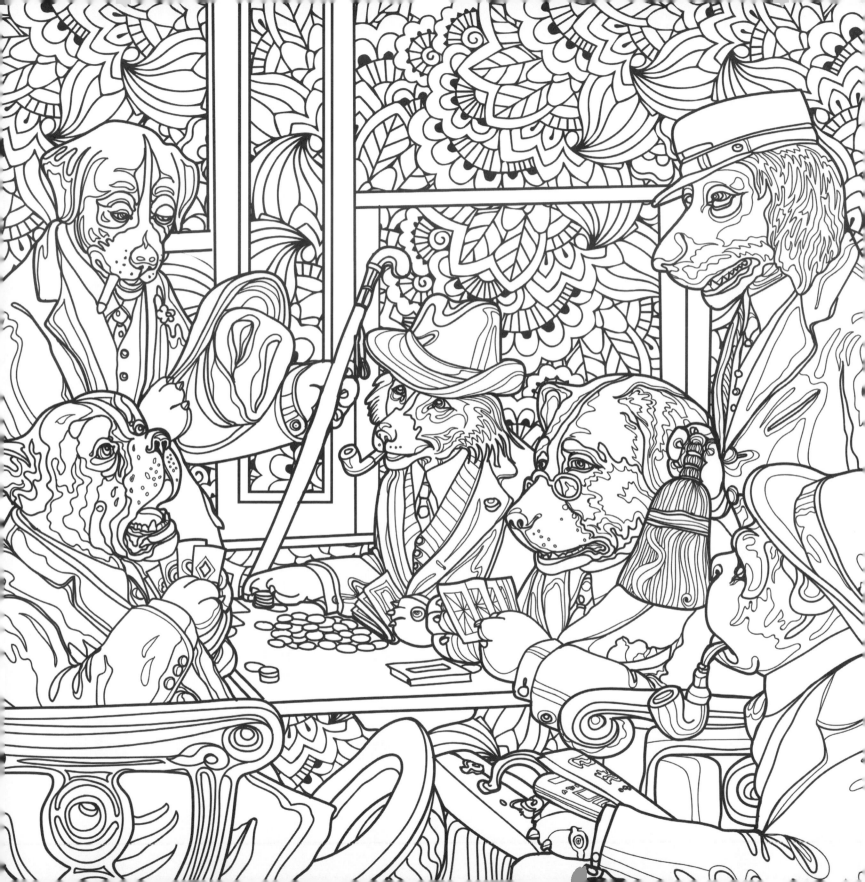

Get quittin' and get happy

This groovy little dude over here is a no smoking zone, the girls all throw him a bone and now he's never alone.

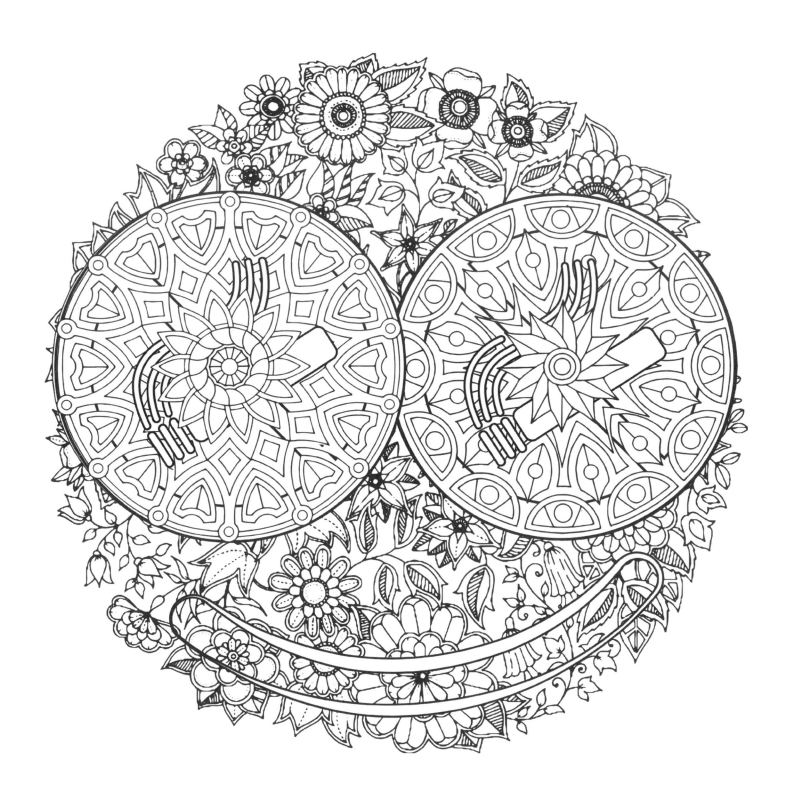

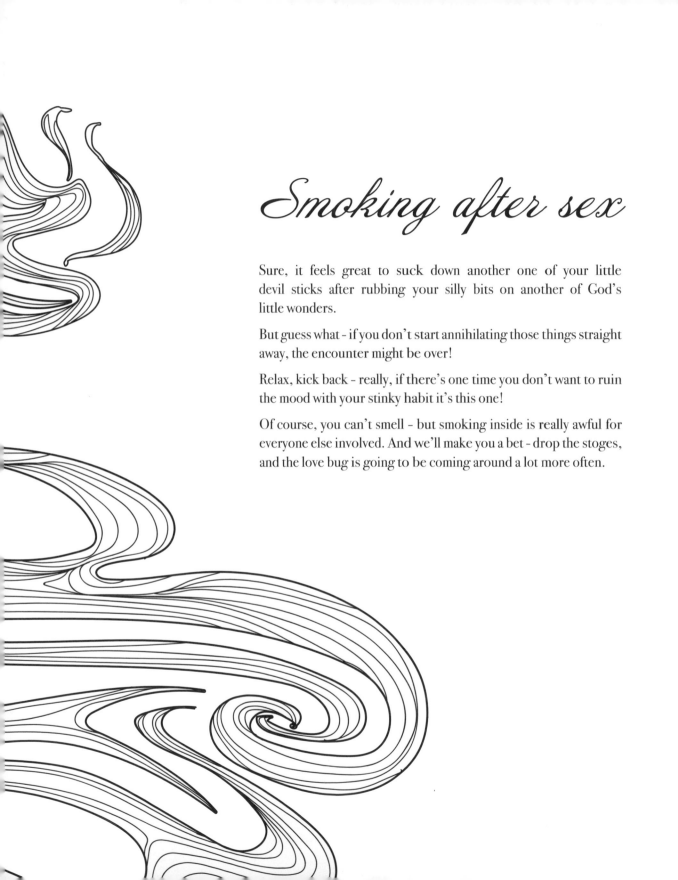

Smoking after sex

Sure, it feels great to suck down another one of your little devil sticks after rubbing your silly bits on another of God's little wonders.

But guess what - if you don't start annihilating those things straight away, the encounter might be over!

Relax, kick back - really, if there's one time you don't want to ruin the mood with your stinky habit it's this one!

Of course, you can't smell - but smoking inside is really awful for everyone else involved. And we'll make you a bet - drop the stoges, and the love bug is going to be coming around a lot more often.

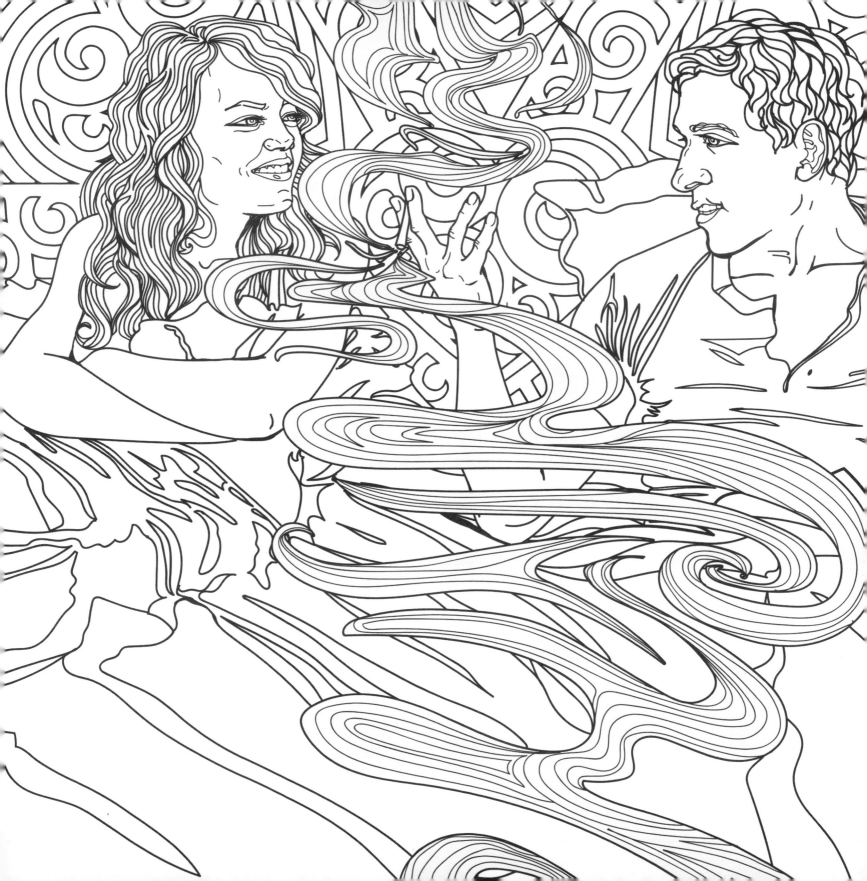

Look at this fella

Pretty unbecoming. And that's before we talk about his hands!

Cigarettes not only ruin our bodies from the inside out, they also throw down heinousness from the outside in.

Exposure to tar through cigarette smoking has potential to stain the fingers and fingernails a hideous yellowish brown colour.

Having a smouldering stick of plant matter between your fingers at temperatures of 400-550*C, and upwards of 700*C whilst being sucked back between your lips, is not an ideal situation for your digits or lips to be in. Blisters, bloody sores and poo-coloured digits are not even the worst of it.

Smoking also goes to town on your blood vessels, particularly in your extremities, negatively effecting dexterity and sensation, as well as limiting blood supply and increasing the likelihood of peripheral vascular disease.

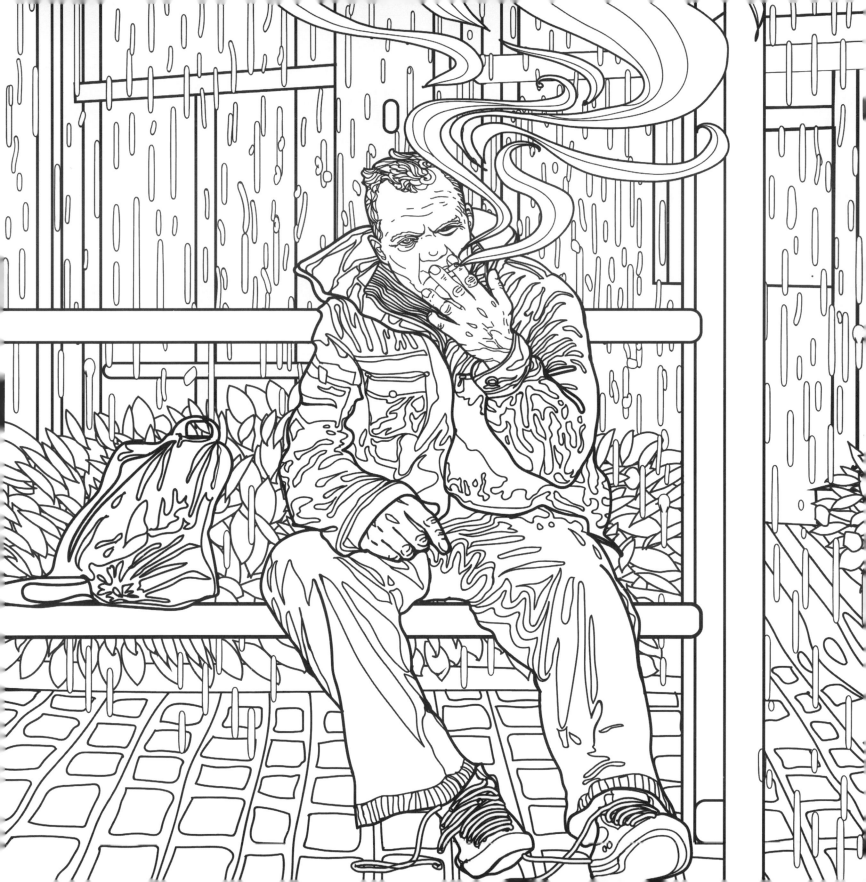

Breathing is better

Thousands of years ago, the Buddha sat underneath a tree, moved his mind with his breath, and pop! Enlightenment! By all reports, the Buddha was a hell of a fella – kind, compassionate, patient, wise. He suffered no more.

Luckily, thanks to the Internet and a bunch of Californian hippies in the '60s, we now have access to this ancient Eastern technique. Boiled down, they say that the ticket to enlightenment is to sit down, with good posture and breathe deeply and regularly. Then, what you want to do is keep this breath going all the time.

Apparently, in Asia, they've been working on this breathing technique for thousands of years.

On the other hand, sometimes we get told to take a breath and count to 10 when we get angry. The irony, of course, is that you already know how to breathe – it's actually instinctive. When your mind wanders, you never stop breathing.

But, you CAN'T breathe. Even if you were trained in Tibetan Buddhism from the age of one, you would still never attain enlightenment. Those horrible sucking noises you make when you run up four stairs don't count.

The real drama is what you've done to your big beautiful shnoz! Breathe in deeply through your nose. Go on, get at it. It's supposed to feel just like breathing through your mouth, but it doesn't – does it? You've had a nose infection for years now!

Smoke irritates the lining of your nose, increases swelling and nasal secretion – this all makes it harder for the big fella to clean itself and that nosey old bitch becomes more susceptible to allergens. Like your classical schoolyard nerd.

The kicker here is that when you meditate, you're supposed to breathe in through your nose, feel the air on the tips of your nostrils, focus on it and breathe out your mouth.

The benefits of meditation are well documented. You become a happy, kind, calm person – which others respond to, generally quite kindly.

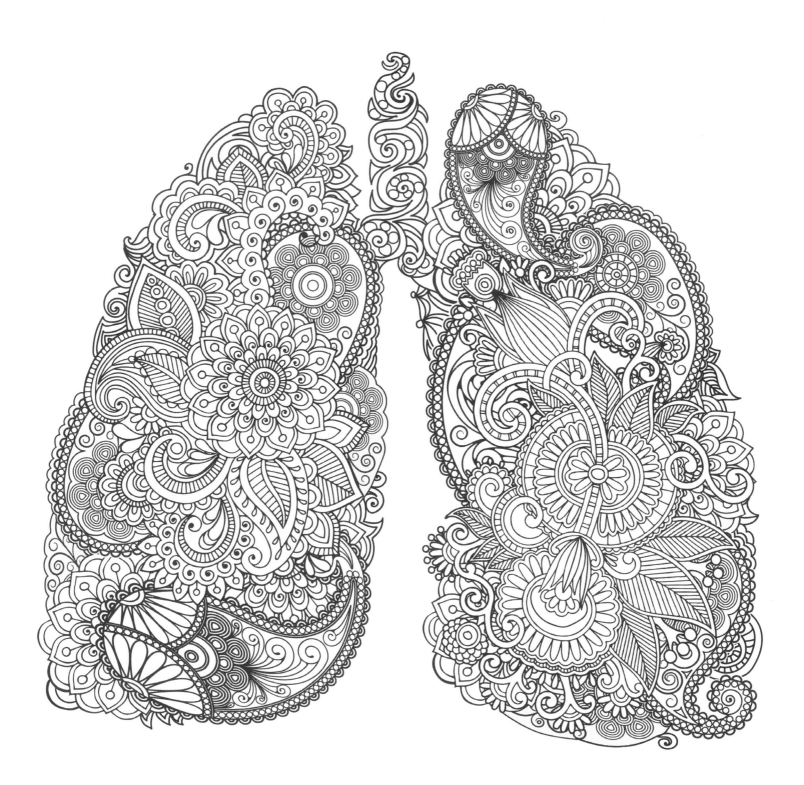

Umm, mmm, coffee and cigarettes

This is another one of your triggers, and it really gets you going in the morning!

Plus, it keeps you regular.

Fun fact - if your body wasn't a disgusting wasteland, you might actually wake up feeling good for once.

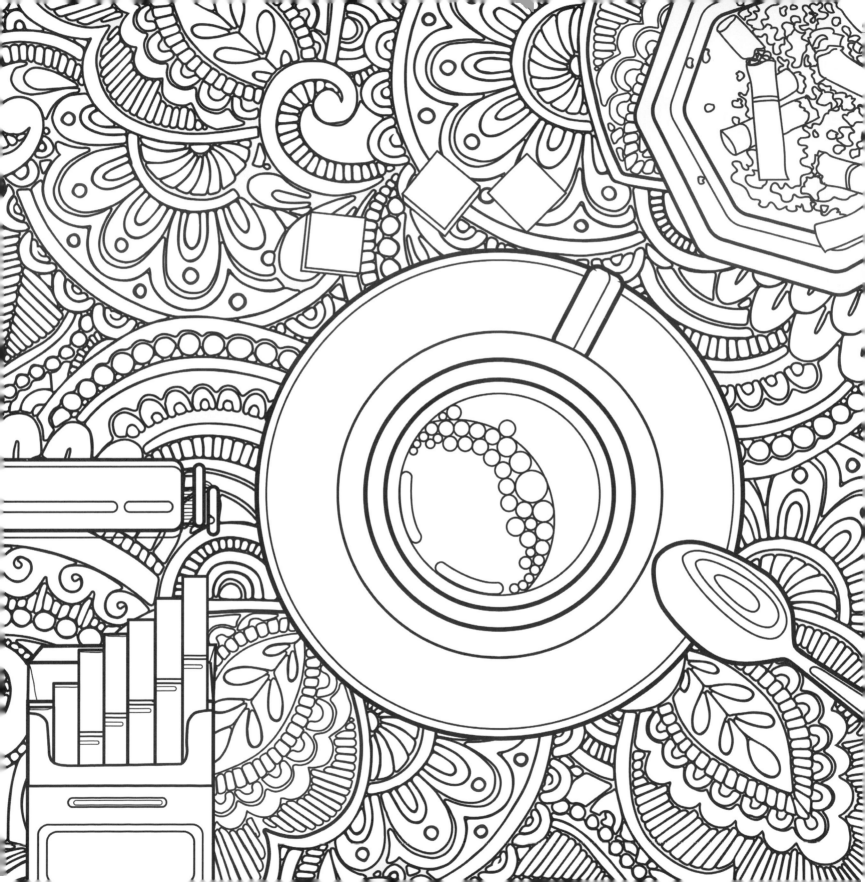

Ain't nobody know what the fuck's in these things!

Why do you eat all organic free range food but light factory farmed chemicals on fire and breathe in the smoke?

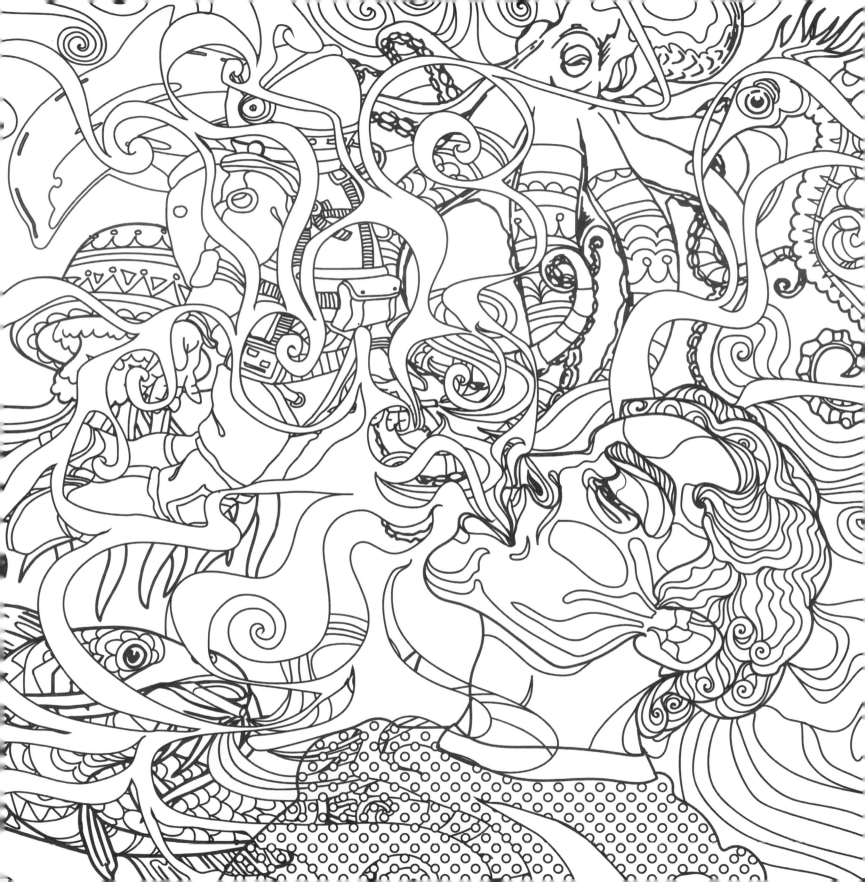

Teeth

A bright smile is the draw card of many attractive people.

A sparkling, not rotten smile, filled with gleaming pearly whites will increase your self esteem as well as improving the likelihood of numerous people of varying sex being keen to get around you and hear your candy chats.

Studies have shown that people are significantly more willing to have sex with people who have nice teeth and pleasant smelling breath.

A way in which to improve the aesthetics of your masticators is to cut out the intake of smoke sticks as the potent mix of CO_2, tar, and only science knows how many other disgusting kinds of junk will only send your teeth straight to brown-town, where the roads are paved in plaque and pot holes.

Smoking and oral hygiene do not go hand in hand so if your teeth are quite brown and smell like a bum, if you're down in the dumps about your bloody gums, if you're sick of your mouth looking like an ass, then tell the next ciggie, "thanks but I'll pass".

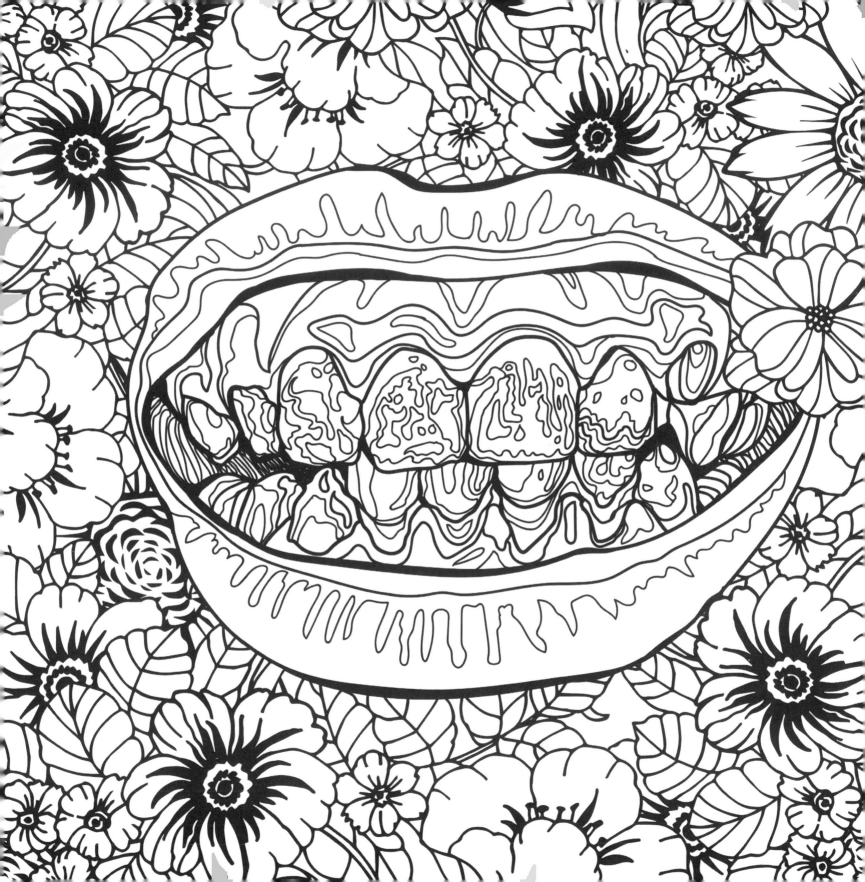

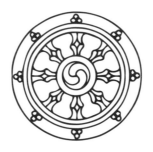

Funky heart

Your heart is for pumping blood and falling in love, not filling with plaque!

Be the heartthrob you can, and let your heart do its thang.

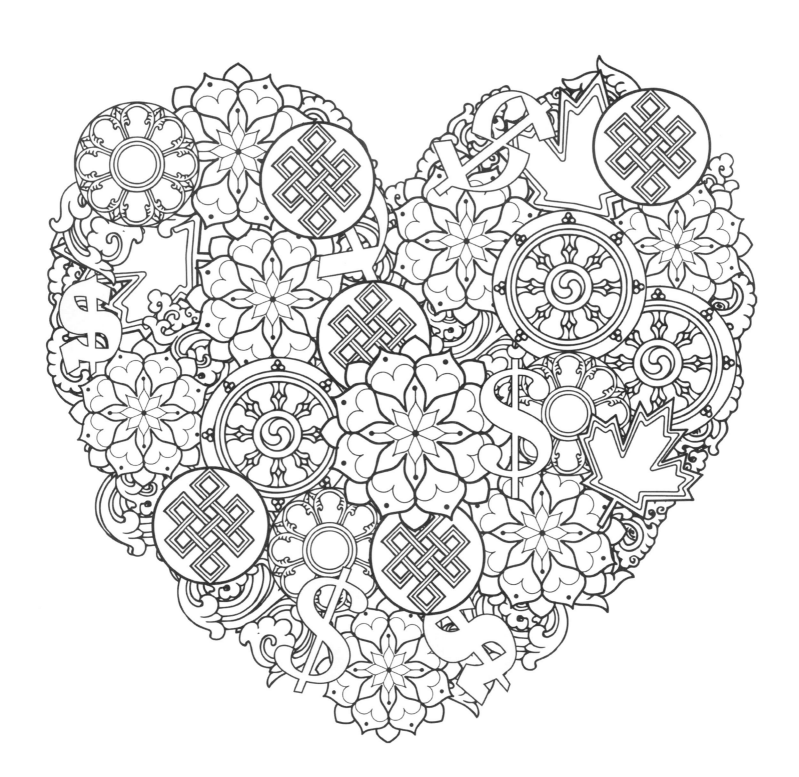

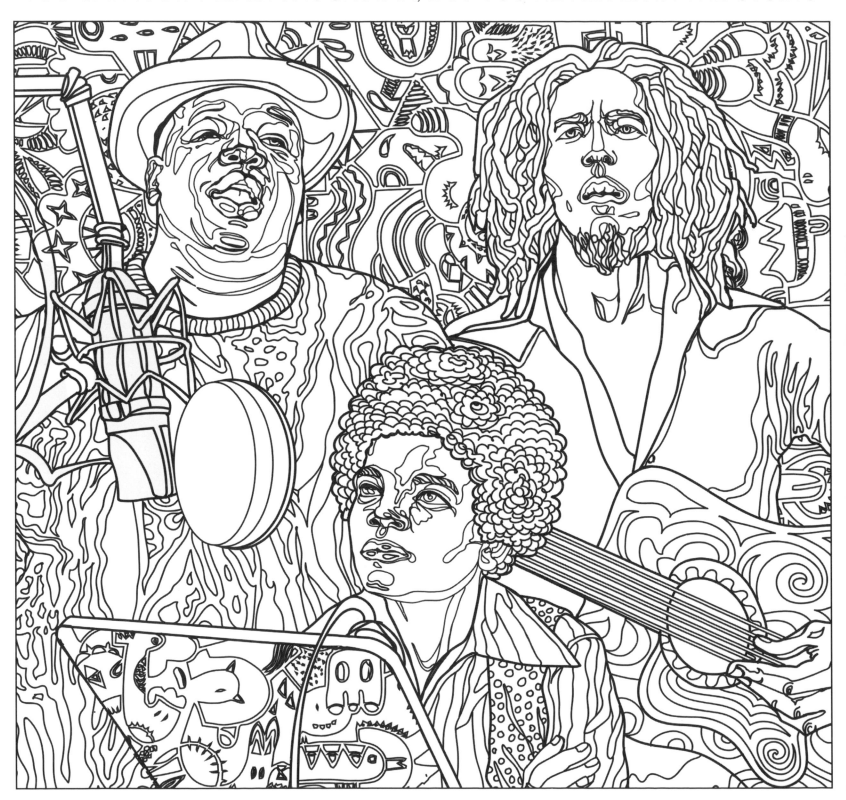

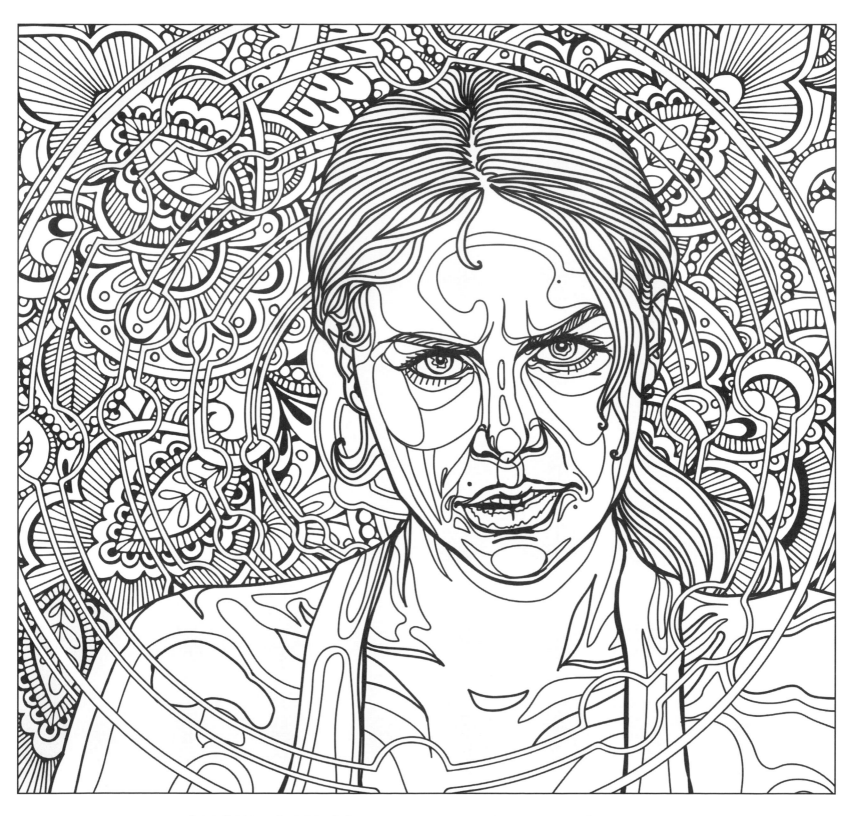

ANGRY STRESSED MIDDLE-AGED WOMAN

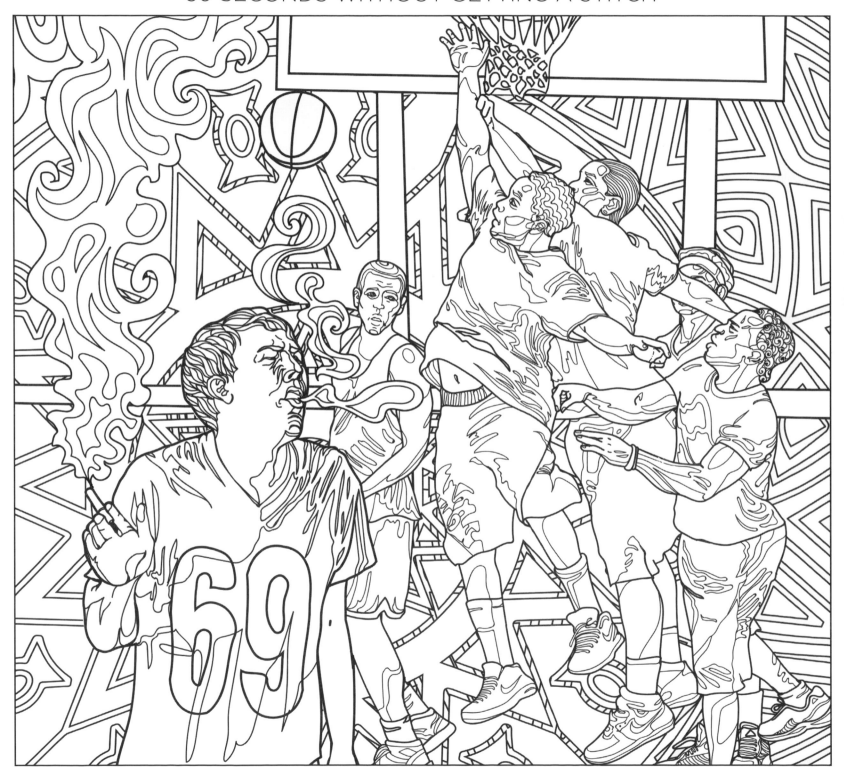

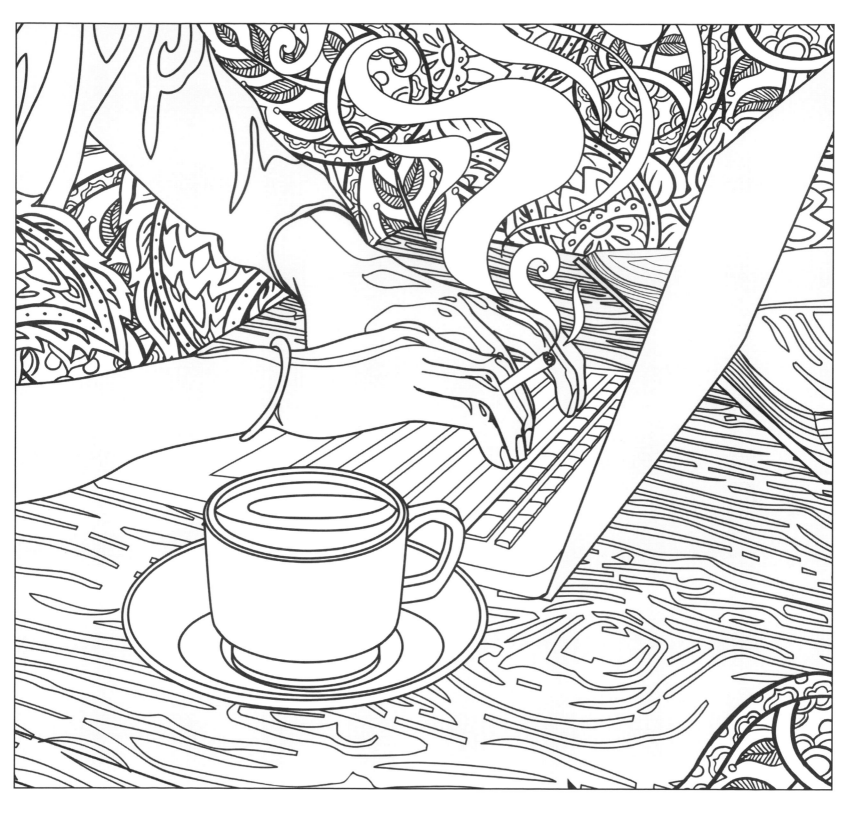

SMOKING HARMS YOUR LAPTOP

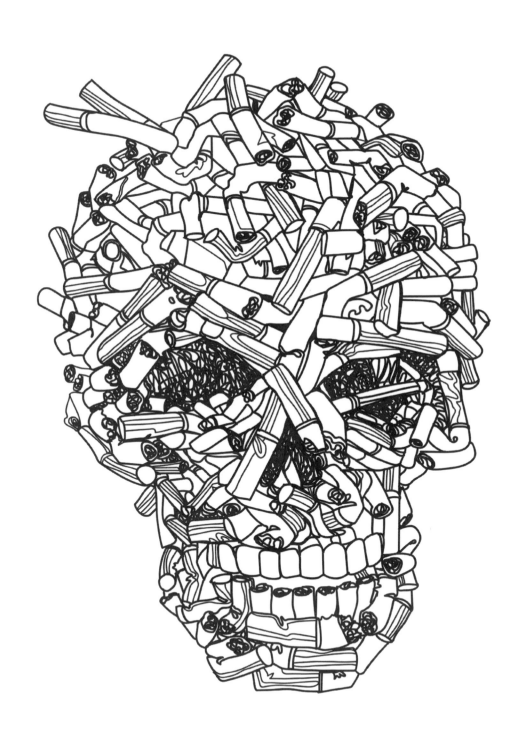

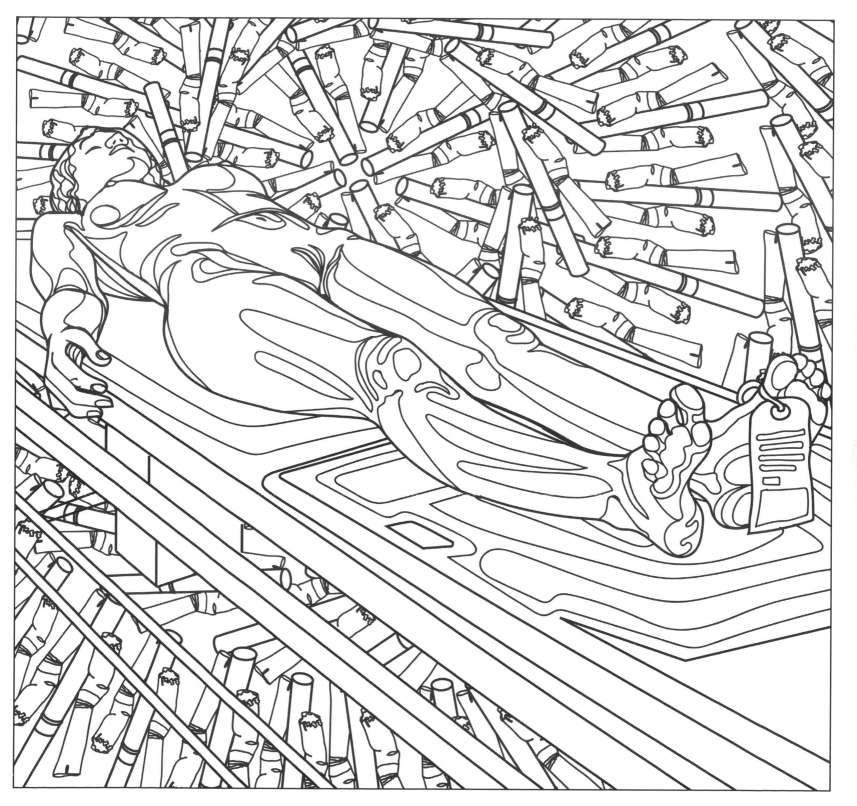

WELCOME TO THE MORGUE, BITCH

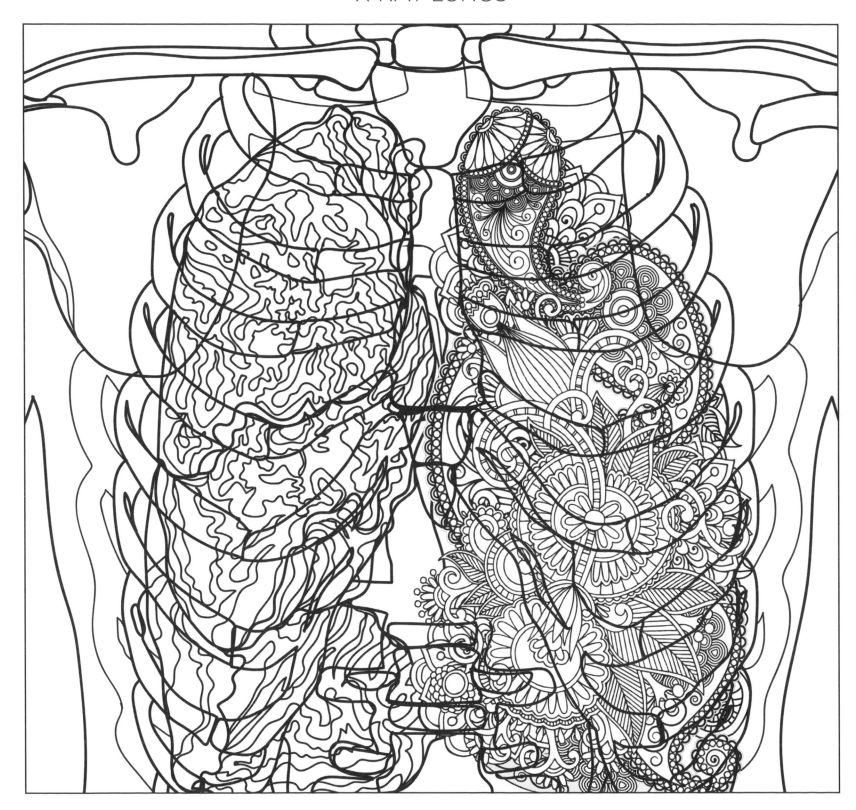

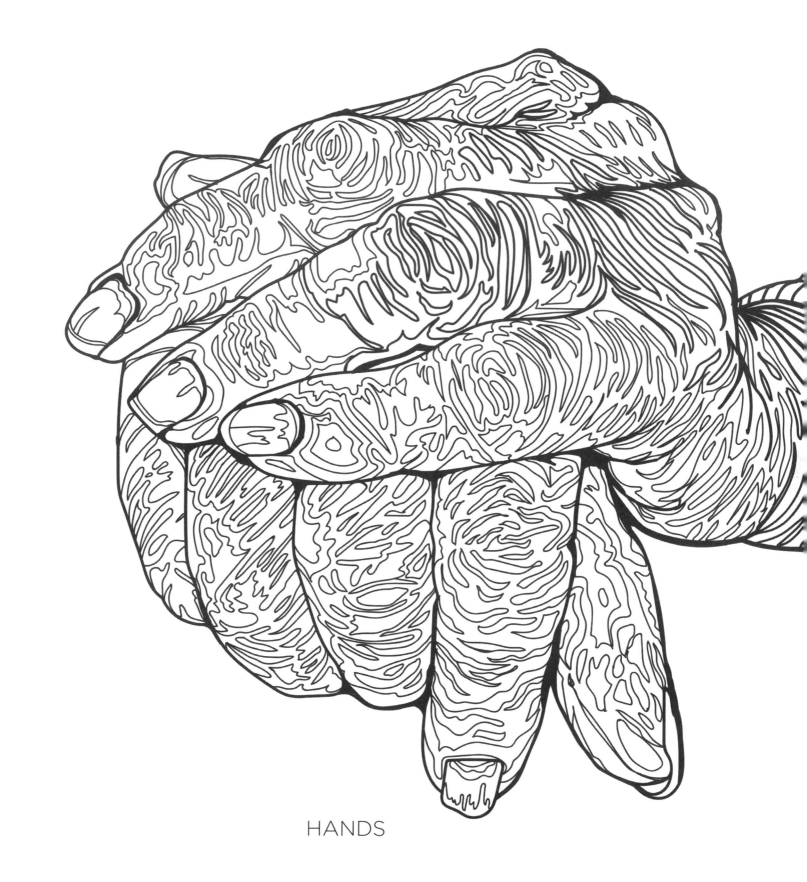

HANDS

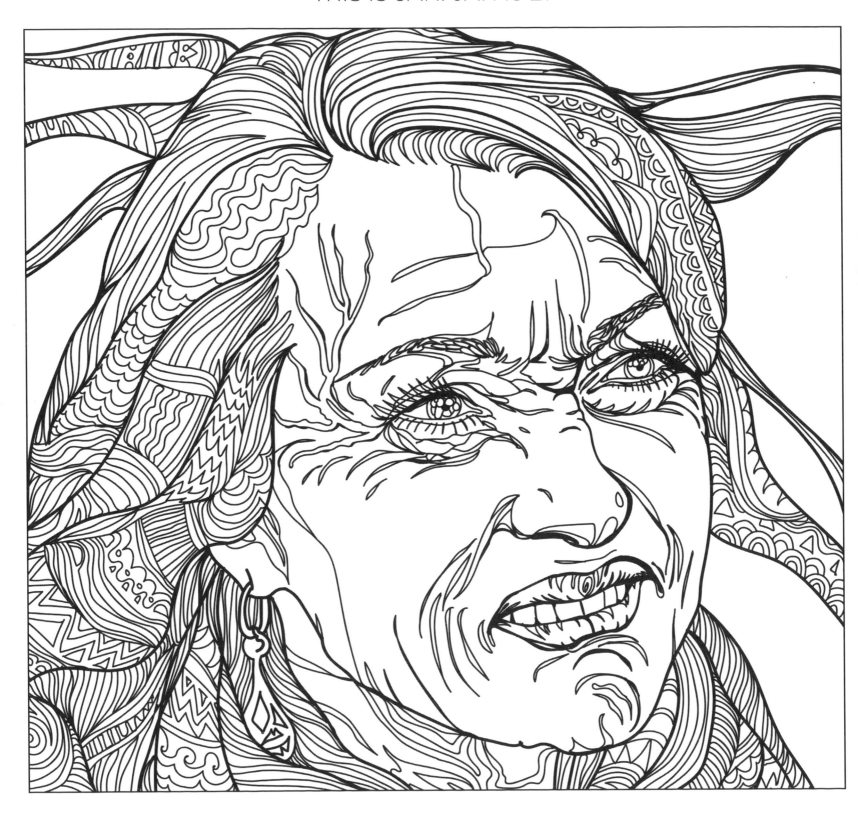

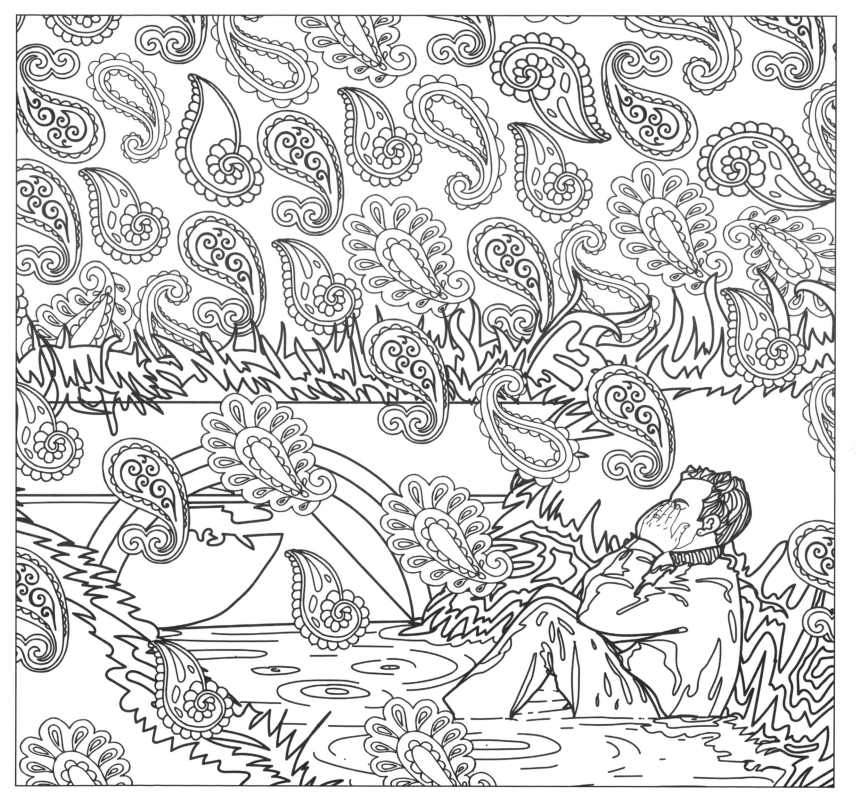

THIS SAD MOTHERFUCKER'S WHOLE FAMILY DIED FROM SMOKING

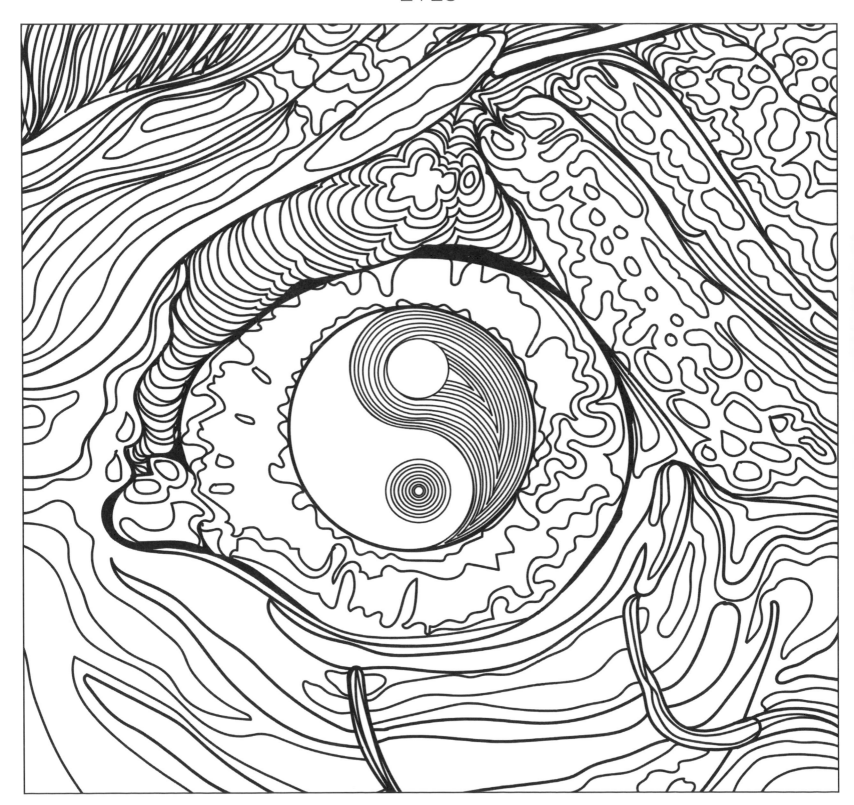

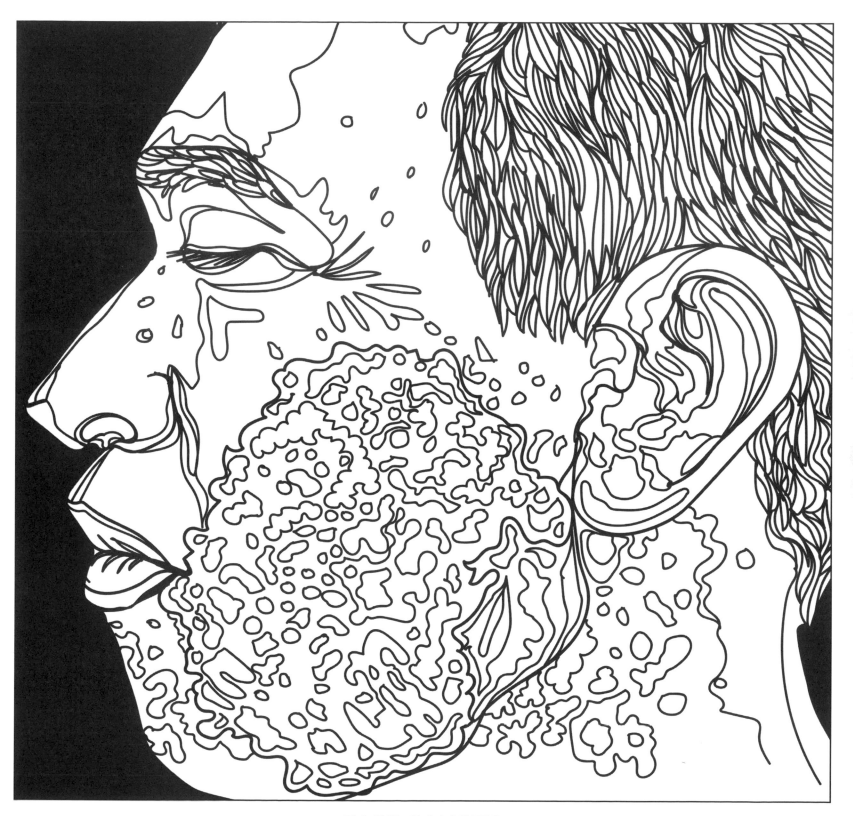

FACE CANCER

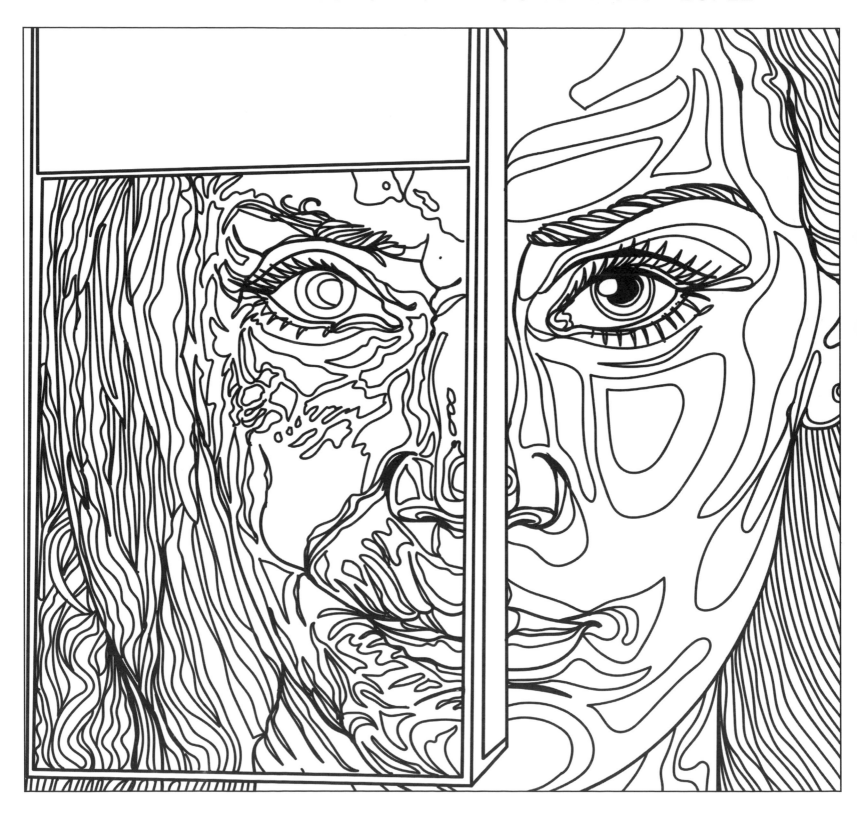

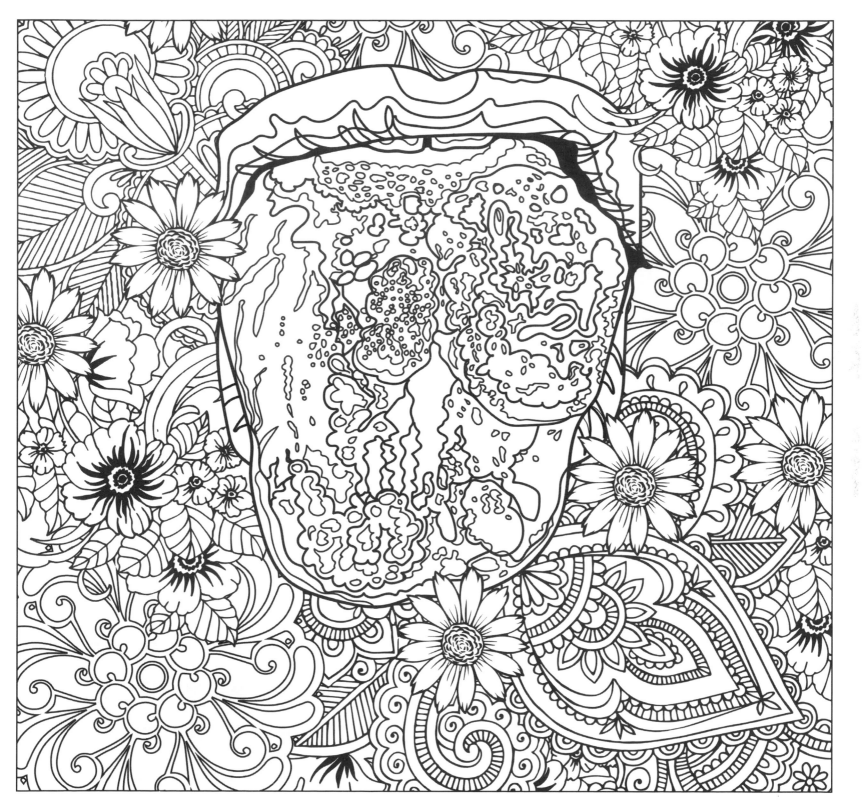

COLOUR IN THE CANCER

Your poor tastebuds

The toxic chemicals you release into your beautiful, love spittin' mouth get right into your tongue and do something lab dorks call "vascularization", which makes your taste buds lose their shape and become flatter. Anywhere else on the body, this would be embarrassing – but luckily your tongue is hidden inside your mouth, and your taste buds are very small.

Smoking cigarettes stuffs your nose up real bad, as well. Smell is a very important factor of tasting food as well.

Why does it matter that smoking dulls your tastebuds?

Interestingly, life is very painful. Humans are a unique animal in that we suffer constantly from a great sense of anxiety that has something to do with farming, industrialisation and globalisation. Eating food is one of the many pleasures available to us to make this suffering a little easier to bear.

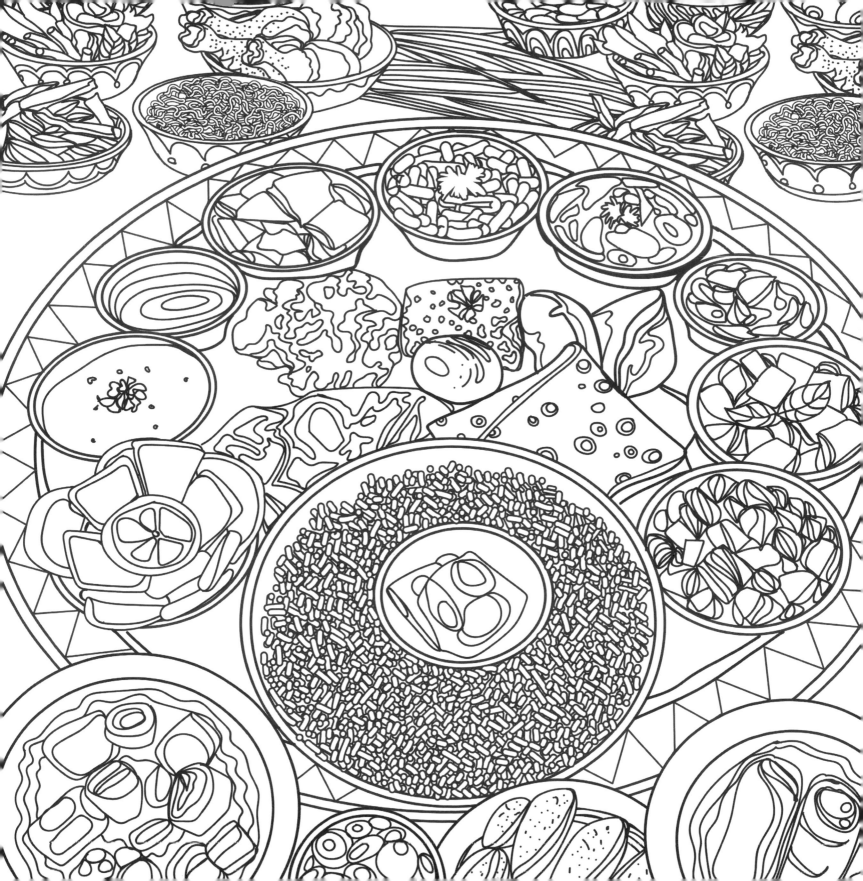

A Scene – 'Couple Fights in a Restaurant'

A Beautiful Girl: Chad, darling, you just must taste this risotto. It's absolutely to die for.

She loads some onto a fork and romantically aeroplanes it into the Smelly Smoker's mouth.

A Smelly Smoker: Oh, Gwen, you know these risottos all just taste like boiled rice!

A Beautiful Girl: I'm sick of this, Chad! It's all the time with you. I work hard, six days a week, just so you can do your crummy little drawings all day long, and all that I want in return is to go to a nice dinner with my lover and have a beautiful meal, enjoying the rich complexities of the flavours of Chef's incredible risotto. And you, you stupid idiot – smoke, smoke, smoke, smoke, smoke. Risotto is incredible, it is delicious. I need a real man.

A Smelly Smoker: But, bab—

A Beautiful Girl: Get out of here, you loser! I hate you and your dumb, flat ugly taste buds!

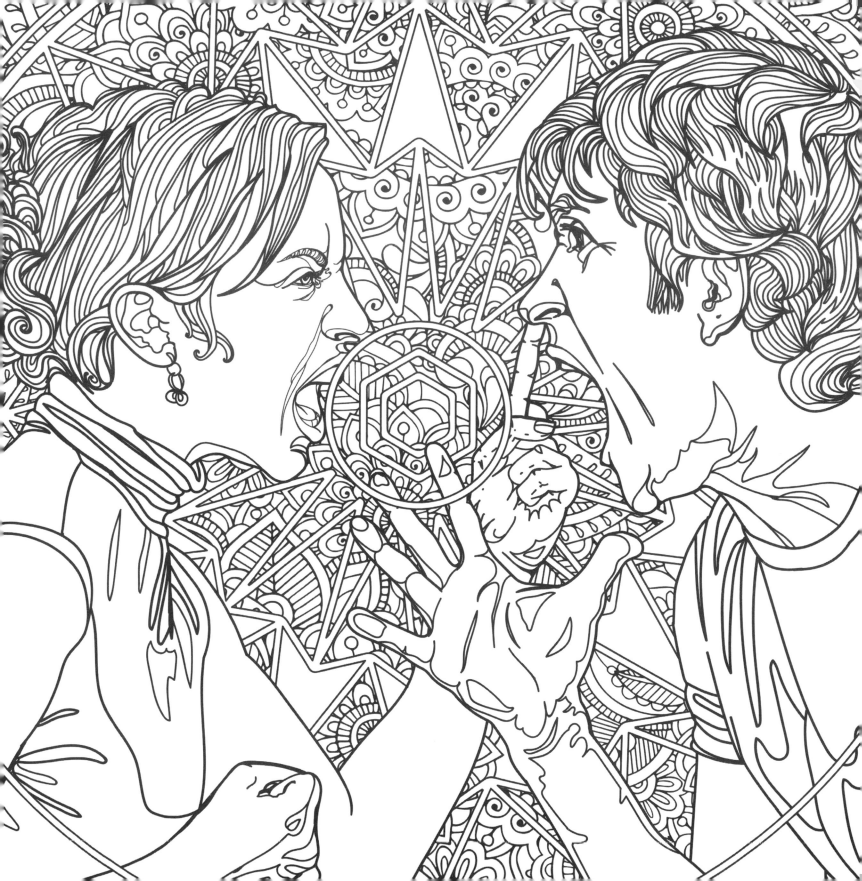

Feet

Do you enjoy comfortably sporting thongs on a hot summers day?

Do you enjoy the benefits of having 10 little piggies transporting you around and maintaining your balance?

Do you have a foot fetish that revolves around sucking toe and lightly nibbling the toe nails and cuticles of your partner?

If you answered yes to any of these questions then chances are you're keen to avoid gangrene in your extremities.

I'll tell you what isn't cute-ical, the fact that smoking can cause peripheral vascular disease.

Smoking limits the blood supply to your feet, hands and other appendages by narrowing and blocking your blood vessels. This means that rich, oxygenated blood doesn't make it round to your fingers and toes putting smokers at significantly greater risk of hideous sores, many of which will take longer to heal without a nourishing blood supply, potentially leading to pain, infection, gangrene and amputation!

So if marketplaces, roast beef and the ability to run all the way home squealing with glee appeals then stop smoking or your little piggies are heading straight to the abattoir.

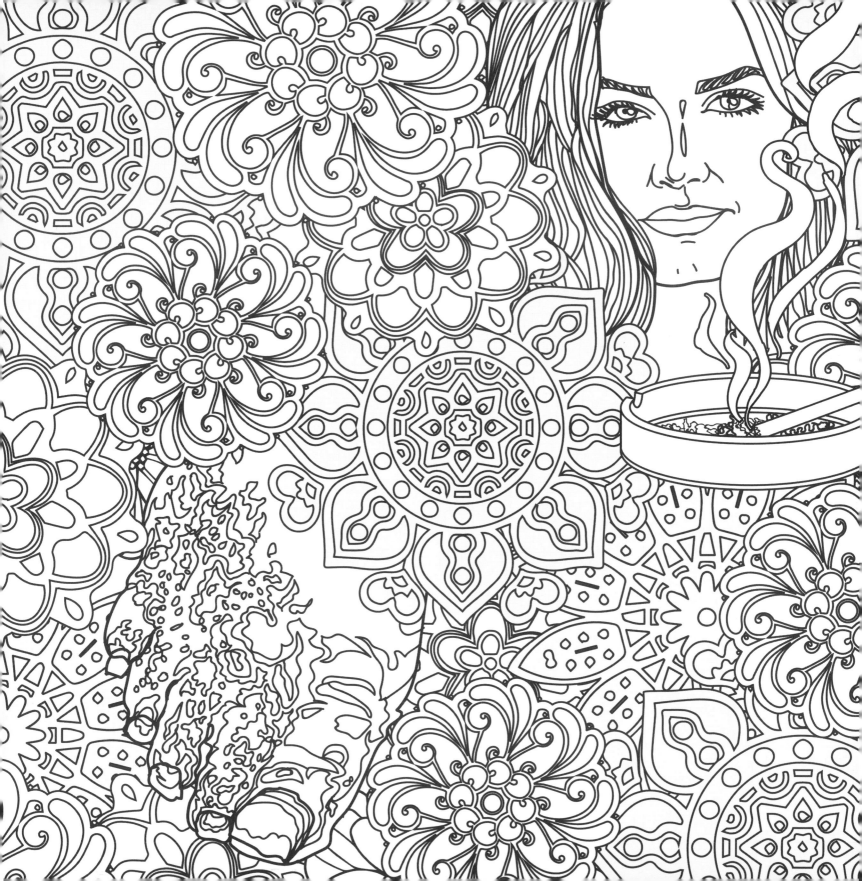

Don't be nervous

Your nervous system is the business. It comes out of that big ol' cerebrum you've got up there that you think you do all your thinking with and spreads out to the rest of the body.

The system consists of the brain, spinal cord and nerves that connect the two and run throughout the body. Electrical impulses are carried from the muscles back to the brain to be analysed, and this constant cycle is how we control everything we do.

Here's what you need to know about what smoking does to your nervous system - it makes you a *sad, dumb bitch.*

Serotonin and dopamine (we know you've heard of these, you pathetic old druggie) are both associated with depression. These are your happiness and excitement chemicals. You mess these up and you become one big ol' sad sack of shit. Staying on the couch, watching Netflix, ignoring your friends' calls, can't find the will to get out of bed, living in a hell dimension that seems impossible to escape, that you will be trapped in forever.

Long-term smoking can have a pretty gnarly impact on your cognitive abilities, too. The neurotransmitters associated with learning, memory, and cognition are all affected by that tasty habit of yours. You're at high risk for dementia, the disease that makes your family hate you before you die. Ciggie munching is also associated with brain matter degeneration and cellular death – and trust us, you need that shit to think! That is all to say, chowing down on smokalokes is making you dumber by the minute.

GABA is the neurotransmitter that is most responsible for your sense of well-being. Smoking trashes it, and raises your levels of anxiety greatly. Your present from smoking - a twitchy, cranky, mean new you.

That could be your life forever, you *sad, dumb, bitch.*

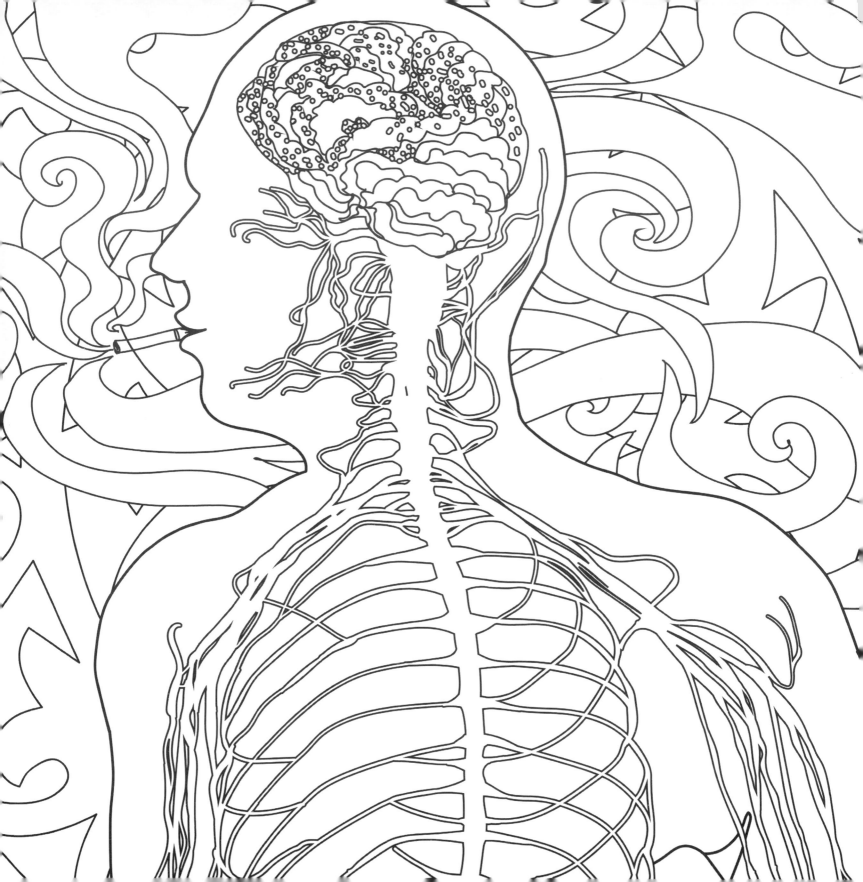

Smoking and your little guy

Smoking damages your blood vessels and gets in the way of proper blood flow. And we all know where blood flow is most important!

Men who don't smoke have harder, stronger erections than those who don't - and they can reach arousal five times faster than their smoking brethren.

Smoking is bad for your sperm, too - maybe due to inflammation in the testicles. Now, inflamed testes sounds like a good thing, but you've got to be careful what you wish for.

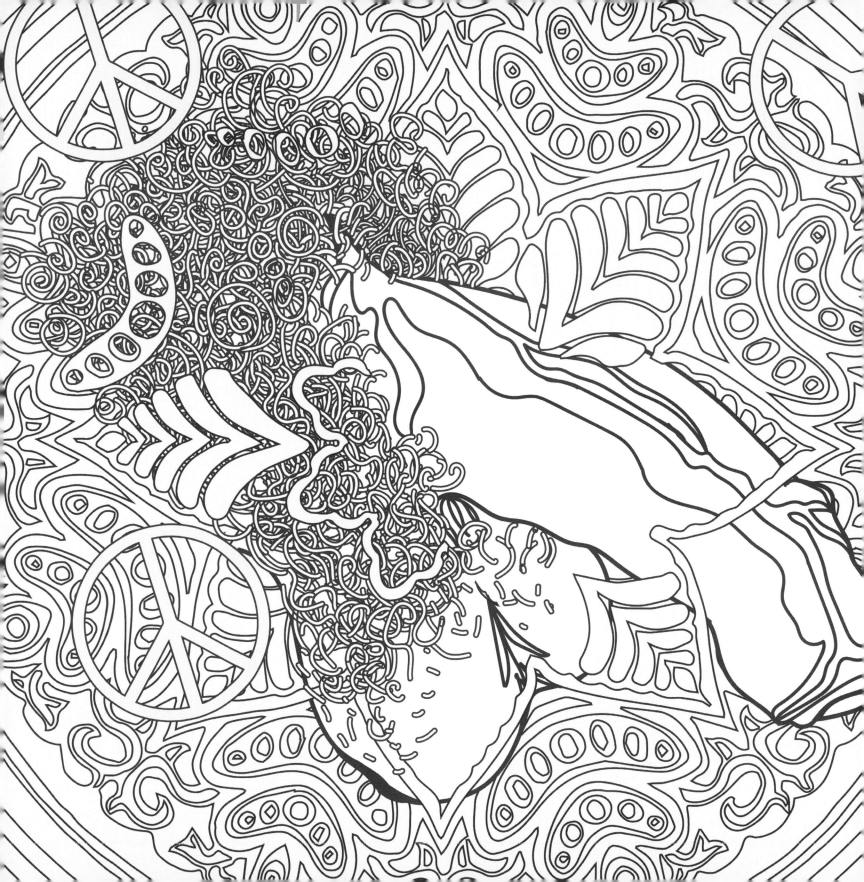

Look at these assholes

Young, in love - jogging. Exercising together in public. Certainly, no one is asking you to act like these people - in fact, we ask that you never, ever do. But that doesn't mean you can't feel the way they feel!

Exercise is an excellent, proven antidote for depression and anxiety - and being depressed and anxious sucks. Exercising releases endocannabinoids stored in the body to make you feel great. Of course, having never done a day's exercise in your life you may be sceptical of this. But, you might recognise the middle of that long word over there as something you have done - *cannabis* - that's right, runner's high is a real thing.

Now drop the darts and go and get it! You'll be grinning like a dope in no time.

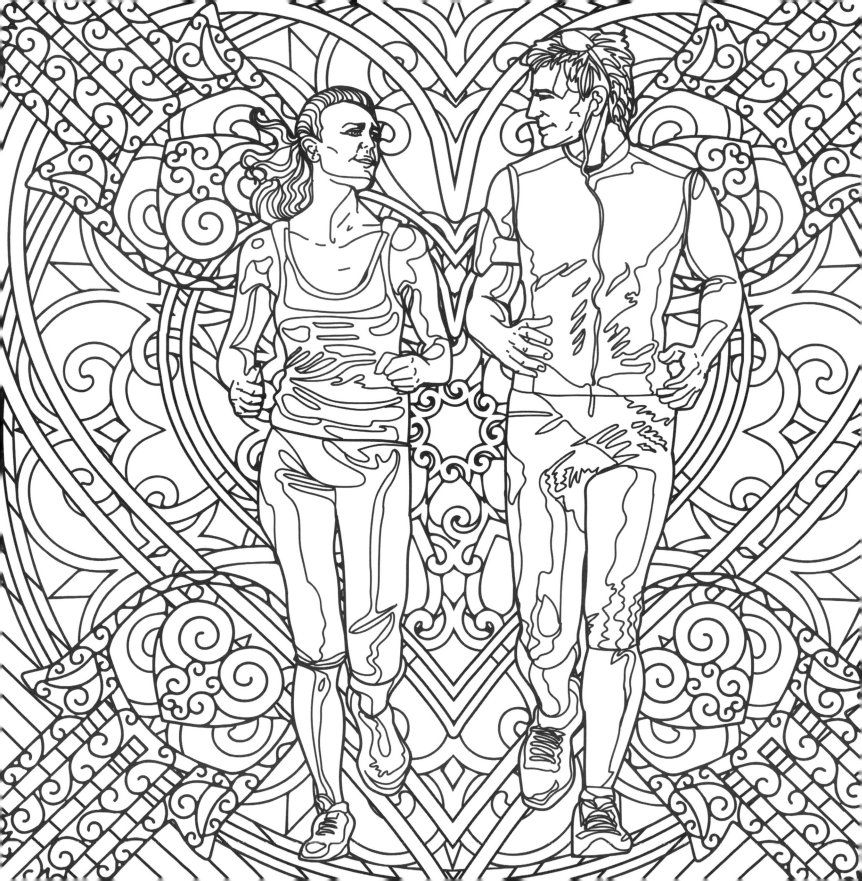

Your heart is responsible for keeping you alive

This is a super scientific diagram of what smoking does to your heart.

Yuck.

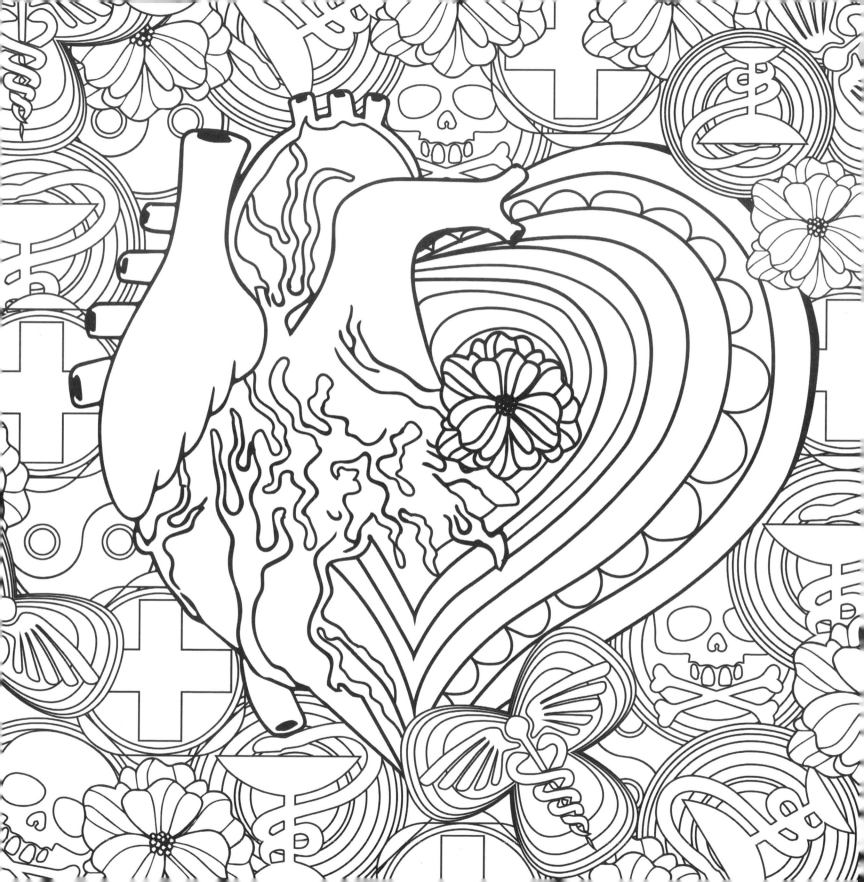

Didn't you see what happened to grandad?

For years, Grandad was a hero. He'd take the kids to the beach, he'd buy 'em desert with a sneaky wink and he'd tell tall stories about all that he got up to back when everything was in black and white and they used coal powered dishwashers. He'd speak about the hearts he broke and left behind, those joyous dances whirled starkly against the austerity and severity of the war, the constant fear of doom.

He taught Josh how to catch a ball and he taught Sally how to throw a punch. He lived a long and full life - a rich and beautiful existence.

But didn't ya see what happened to Grandad? When he spent all those years moving around painfully with that walker, and when he couldn't even do that anymore. When you could hardly hear his voice as his eyes sparkled to tell a story, when he broke into coughing fits that wouldn't stop for hours, and hours. Didn't ya see Grandad on that bed, moving around, barely conscious, writhing in pain?

Didn't you see your Mum crying when her Dad didn't know where he was? When he thought it was 1943 and he was buying Celia her first drink? Didn't you see how scared he looked when he realised he was in the hospital?

Didn't you see Sally, crying at the foot of his bed, when we all knew it was going to end? Didn't you see your Grandad die in front of your eyes and how awful it was for everyone you loved?

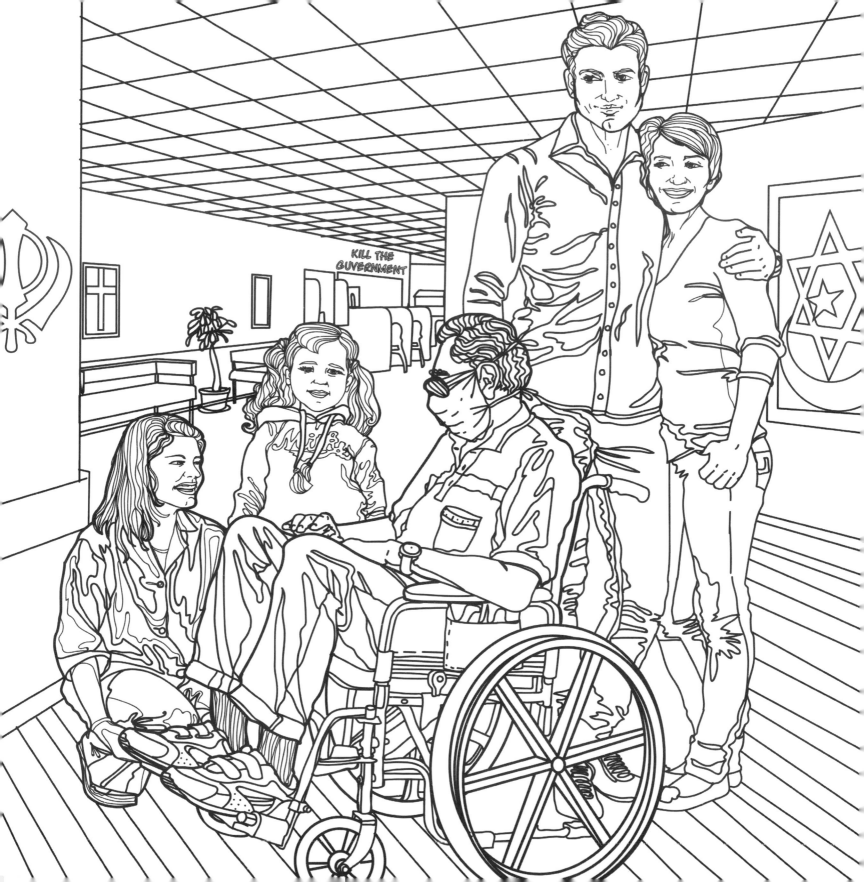

Hey pal, do you like walking?

This is your spine. He does the hard yards, keeping you up and moving.

Smoking cigarettes causes hardening of the arteries which decreases blood supply to areas fed by small blood vessels.

Discs in the spine don't have their own blood supply and rely on the nutrients of the surrounding tissues. They can starve for oxygen and other nutrients.

Cigarettes make degenerative spinal problems worse, and your every day ability to move could be at risk!

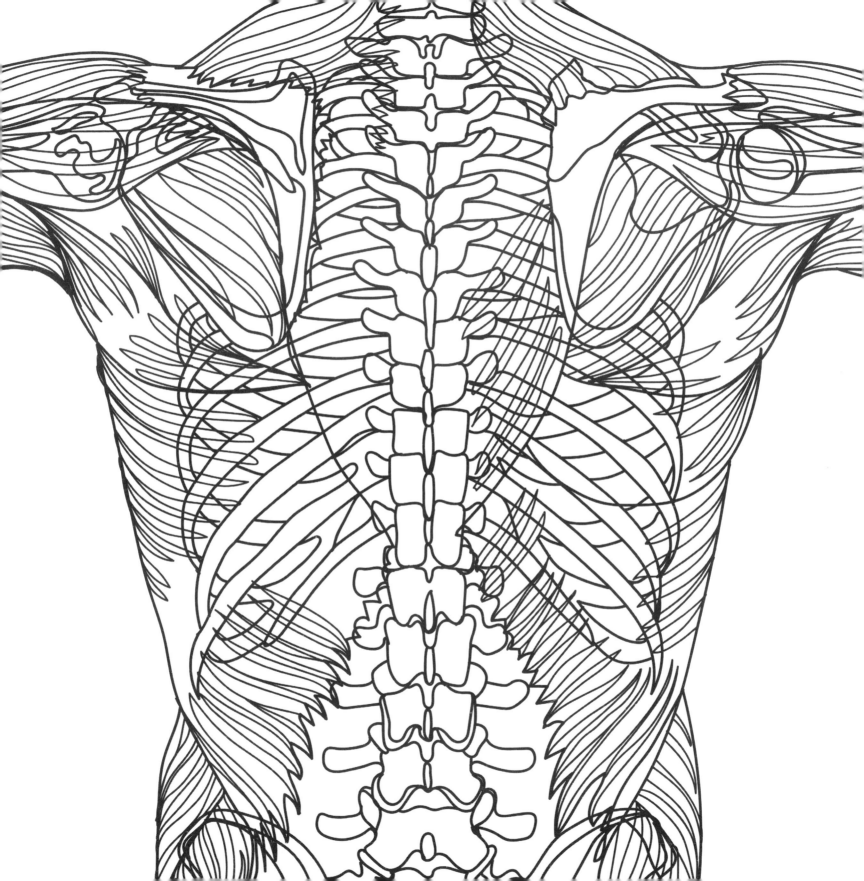

The hole in your throat

You've seen it on TV, you've even seen it in real life. People with a hole in their throat.

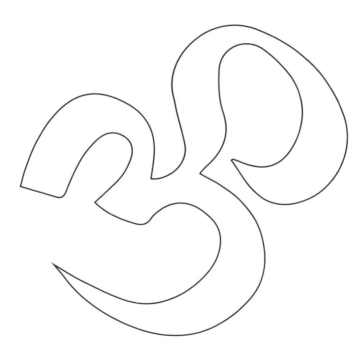

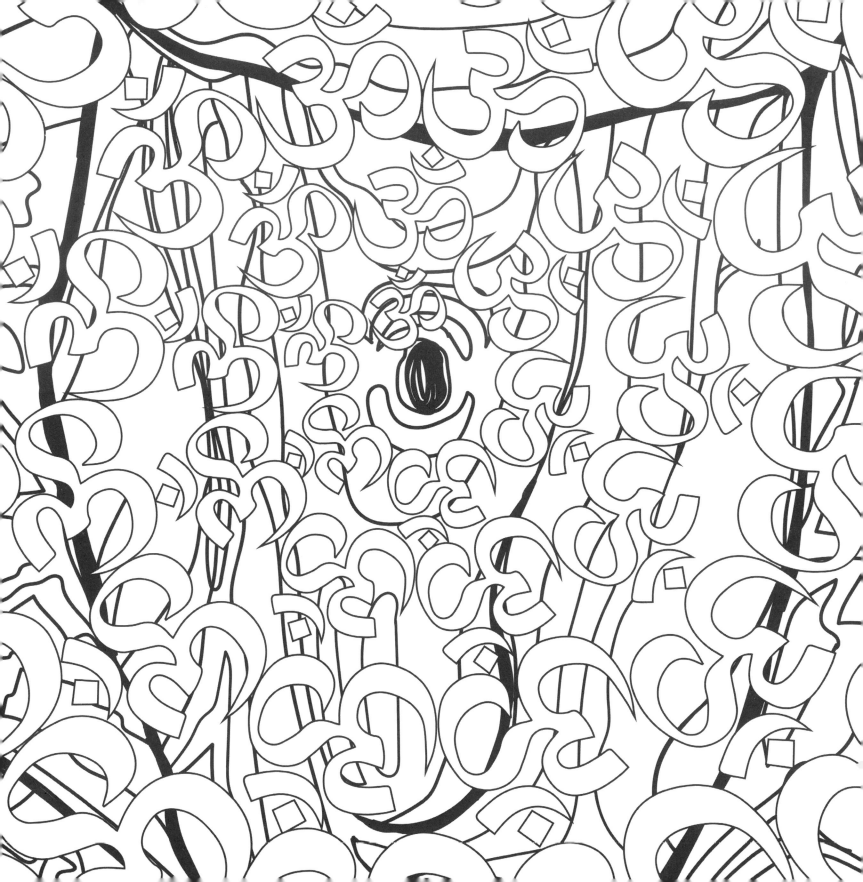

Check out Doctor Hunk!

Sure, you might think that by continuing to smoke you're going to be running into beautiful ladies and gentleman like this all the time.

But get a grip, Doctor Handsome isn't in the hospital to crack onto some pock-marked toothless old hag. He thinks you're pathetic, and a waste of the precious scarce medical resources - you do this to yourself, so why don't you just get some self control and make Doctor Wonderful a happy man?

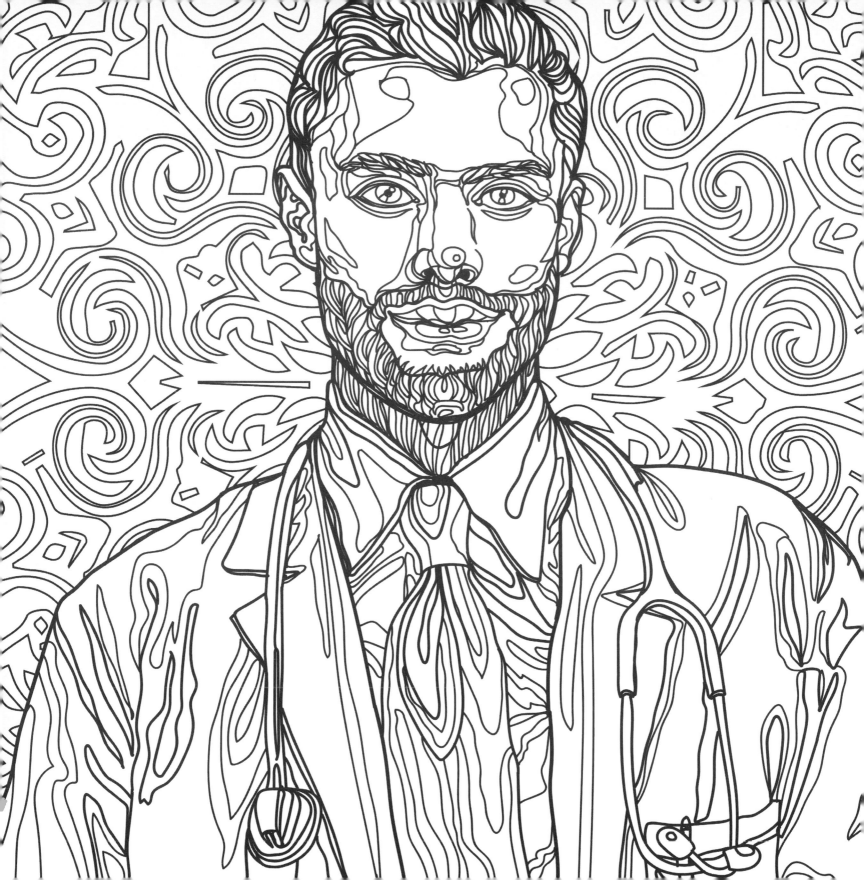

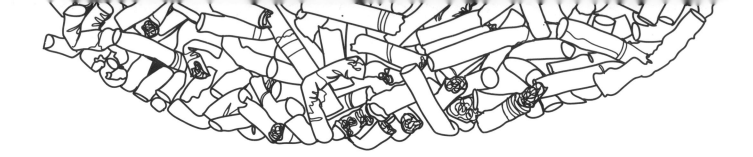

You smell like an ashtray

Nobody has ever said "hmm that ash-tray smells delicious" so it should be abundantly clear that the stank emanating from your person after a cigarette would not be any different.

If you remain oblivious to the fact that you smell like a dead animal's anus after a cigarette that is because smoking not only makes you smell like said anus, but also significantly dulls your own sense of smell.

Smoke particles invade the fibres of your clothes, the essence of your breath and soaks into your hair.

Even smokers would attest to not finding assholes, dead animals and musk and muted stench particularly appealing.

Similarly to how applying deodorant to a BO infested armpit only exacerbates the pong, no amount of cologne, perfume, or body spray can completely eradicate the persistent stench of cigarette smoke.

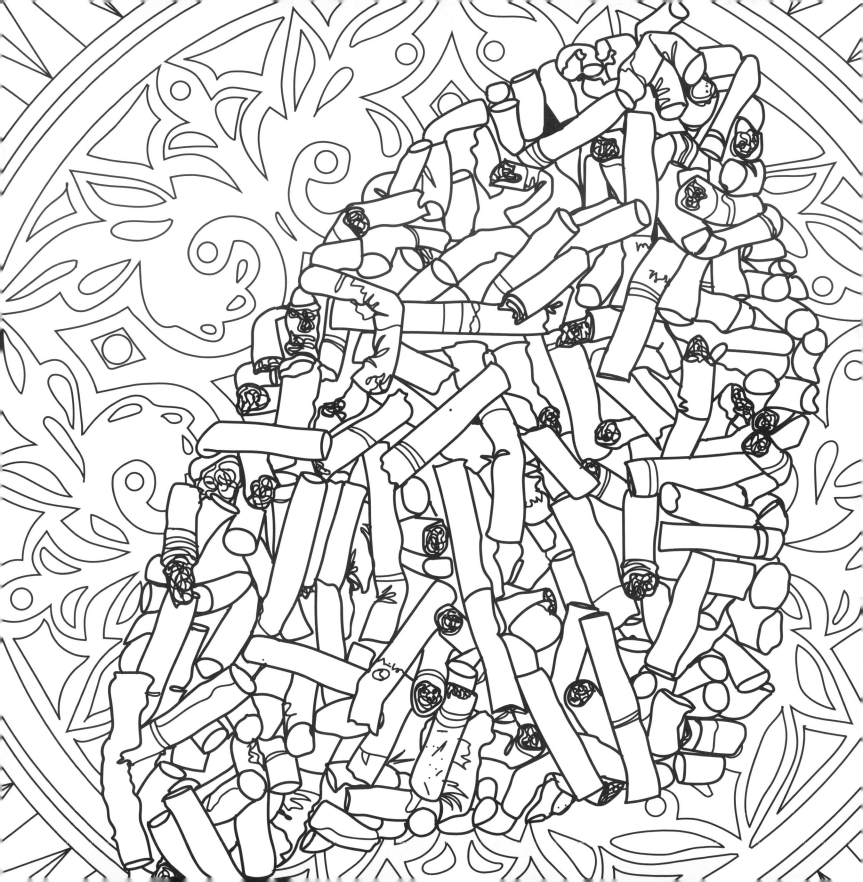

Smoking doubles your risk of stroke

And that's fine if you're not worried about having one side of your body permanently paralysed.

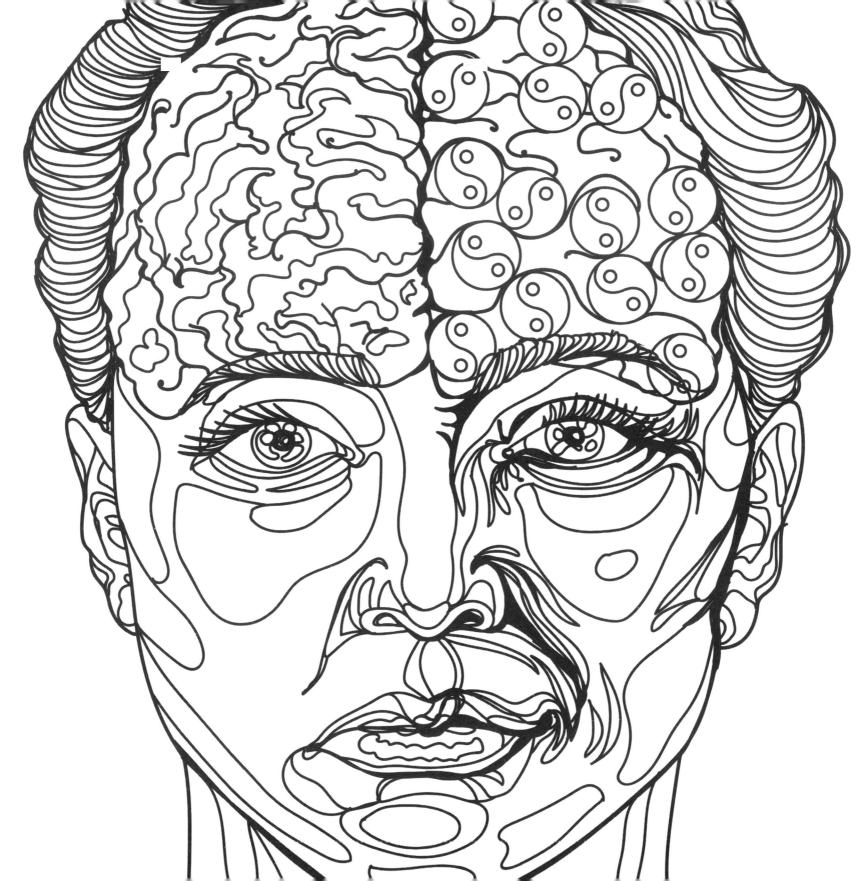

Look at this monster

You've seen 'em, driving along the highway, chain-smoking in the car with the little Brad while they both gulp down 40oz. Coca Colas.

Sure, you don't have kids now - but you will. Probably with the other gross, overweight, sad, angry person you met hiding out the back of Jessica's wedding suckling on a nail. And then, bam - before you know it - you're just another one of these animals, shoving disease down their own kids' throat.

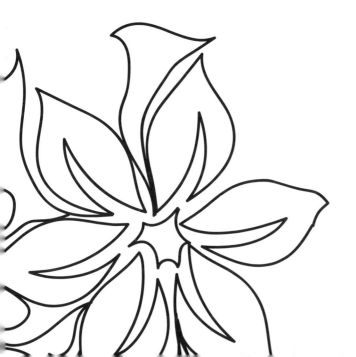

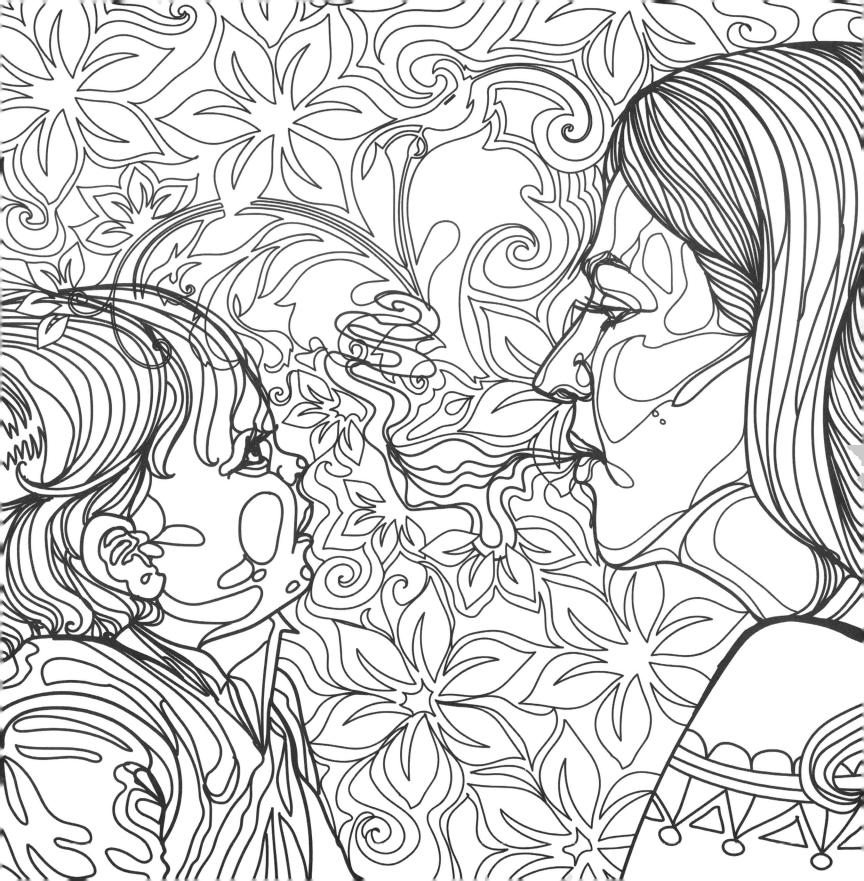

Draw your own sad lungs

Draw your own coughing fit

Draw a hat smoking a cigarette

Draw your own funeral

The end.